GUIDELINES TO GYNAECOLOGY

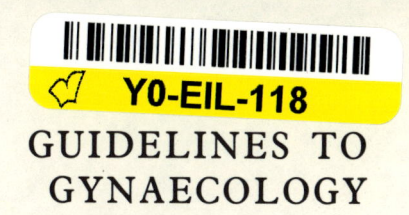

GUIDELINES TO GYNAECOLOGY

Michael D. Read
MB ChB FRCS(Ed) MRCOG
Senior Registrar in
Obstetrics and Gynaecology
North-West Regional Health Authority

Stuart Mellor
MB ChB MRCOG
Consultant Obstetrician
and Gynaecologist
North Manchester General Hospital

Blackwell Scientific Publications
Oxford London Edinburgh
Boston Melbourne

© 1982 by
Blackwell Scientific Publications
Editorial offices:
Osney Mead, Oxford OX2 0EL
8 John Street, London WC1N 2ES
9 Forrest Road, Edinburgh EH1 2QH
52 Beacon Street, Boston,
   Massachusetts 02108, USA
99 Barry Street, Carlton, Victoria 3053
   Australia

All rights reserved. No part of this publication may be reproduced, stored in a retrieval system, or transmitted, in any form or by any means, electronic, mechanical, photocopying, recording or otherwise without the prior permission of the copyright owner

First published 1982

Set by Southline Press, Ferring, W. Sussex
Printed and bound in Great Britain by Billing & Sons Ltd., Worcester

DISTRIBUTORS

USA
   Blackwell Mosby Book Distributors
   11830 Westline Industrial Drive
   St Louis, Missouri 63141

Canada
   Blackwell Mosby Book Distributors
   120 Melford Drive, Scarborough
   Ontario M1B 2X4

Australia
   Blackwell Scientific Book
   Distributors
   214 Berkeley Street, Carlton
   Victoria 3053

British Library
Cataloguing in Publication Data

Read, Michael D.
   Guidelines to gynaecology.
   1. Gynaecology 2. Obstetrics
   I. Title II. Mellor, Stuart
   618   RG101

   ISBN 0-632-009322

Contents

Preface, vii
How to Use this Book, ix

Gynaecological History-Taking, 1
Gynaecological Examination, 3
Gynaecological Emergencies, 5

1. SPECIFIC CONDITIONS
   Abortion, 11
   Pelvic Pain, 17
   Low Back Pain, 19
   Pelvic Masses, 21
   Amenorrhoea, 25
   Post-Menopausal Bleeding, 29
   Heavy or Irregular Menstruation, 33
   Dysmenorrhoea, 37
   Dyspareunia, 41
   Pruritus Vulvae, 43
   Vaginal Discharge, 49
   Cytology of the Female Genital Tract, 53
   Abnormal Cervical Cytology, 55
   Subfertility — Female, 61
   Subfertility — Male, 65
   Urinary Symptoms, 69

Continued overleaf

2. GENERAL TOPICS
Hormone Therapy in Gynaecology, 77
Drugs in Gynaecology, 87
Contraception, 97
Gynaecological Operations — Practical Aspects, 109

Index, 119

Preface

To the newly appointed Senior House Officer, obstetrics and gynaecology is unfamiliar. Many aspects differ from the experience gained (often the hard way) in medicine and surgery. Not only is there a whole new range of conditions and disorders to learn about but also new practical techniques to master. It is not surprising, therefore, that the first few weeks can be a hectic and bewildering experience for the newcomer as he struggles to master the basic ground rules and 'building blocks' of the specialty. His lot is made no lighter by the heavy workload so often encountered, and although he may obtain invaluable guidance and help from more experienced colleagues and read around the subject in the standard textbooks, it is far from easy to develop a practical knowledge and understanding of the various conditions encountered and how they are managed.

This book is designed to give practical guidelines in the management of the more common conditions presenting in the clinics and on the wards. The emphasis is on a step by step approach to diagnosis and management and thus, it is believed, it will complement the more traditional approach of the standard textbook. It is not intended that this brief guide should be regarded as a substitute for either the textbook or practical experience. It therefore deliberately omits descriptions of practical procedures such as D&Cs, therapeutic abortions, and sterilisation. These can be read from larger works but are better learned by instruction and close supervision.

In the interests of clarity and, we hope, easy comprehension it has been necessary to adopt a simple, non-controversial approach. Whilst we appreciate that there are different schools of thought on many of the subjects dealt with, we believe that the information is presented in a form appropriate to the inexperienced newcomer to this interesting and rewarding speciality.

How to Use this Book

The first part of this book consists of step by step flowcharts describing the sequential stages in arriving at the diagnosis of a particular condition and its subsequent management. Each flowchart covers one commonly encountered topic and is accompanied by a series of explanatory notes. In order to achieve our aim — of easy comprehension — the notes present an approach representing the consensus of current opinion rather than the arguments in either direction, which may be obtained from the reference books and journals.

The second part contains advice and information about more general topics, including details of drugs and hormone preparations with the more usual treatment regimes.

It is hoped that this book will go some way to clearing the mists of confusion and help you to *understand* the conditions you meet, and that this basic understanding will lead to an even better service for the patient. Perhaps you may even begin to enjoy gynaecology!

GYNAECOLOGICAL HISTORY-TAKING

It is always important to remember that you are dealing with a patient as a whole person and not to restrict your attention to the pelvis. It is not uncommon for patients to attend the gynaecological out-patient clinic complaining of what turns out to be a local manifestation of a generalised medical disorder. A *full history* should therefore be elicited, allowing the patient to use her own words as far as possible and to take her own time. Many patients are embarrassed and their presenting complaint may not in fact be the problem which is troubling them most. A sympathetic and professional approach will be well rewarded, while specific points in the history may be clarified by tactfully posed, direct questions. In view of the likely embarrassment of the patient, it is of utmost importance that the history is taken in complete privacy, not in the open clinic.

Many departments make use of the pre-printed pro-forma history sheets which ensures that the important details are always recorded and that there is a uniformity of presentation.

When you have dealt with the presenting complaint, it is important to elicit an accurate *menstrual history*, beginning with the date of the last normal menstrual period. The menarche is important when dealing with infertility, amenorrhoea, and adolescent menstrual irregularities. Details of the menstrual cycle are recorded in a fractional notation with the duration of the loss as the numerator and the cycle length (from first day of a period to the first day of the next period) as the denominator. In patients with an irregular cycle it is usual to record the shortest and longest cycles over the previous six months.

The amount of the loss is very subjective but if clots are present, if the patient is unable to control the flow with tampons alone, or she uses more than 24 pads per period, it is reasonable to assume the loss is heavy. The occurrence of *irregular* bleeding per vaginam, such as inter-menstrual, post-coital or post-menopausal bleeding, is very important. This pattern of bleeding which is unrelated to menstruation may be due to an underlying malignancy. Typical examples are post-coital bleeding, which suggests a local lesion such as carcinoma of the cervix or vagina, or post-menopausal bleeding which requires exclusion of a higher lesion such as carcinoma of the endometrium. If there is any pain associated with the periods it is important to elicit the time of onset in relation to the menstrual flow and whether it eases or worsens with the flow. (These details may help to differentiate between primary and secondary dysmenorrhoea, pelvic inflammatory disease and endometriosis.) The nature, site and radiation of the pain are also important.

The *obstetric history* is of relevance in many conditions, including sub-fertility, habitual abortion, carcinoma of the cervix, and genital prolapse. Details of *all* pregnancies and their outcome should be recorded, along with any complications.

Urinary symptoms are not uncommon presenting complaints in the gynaecological clinic and it is important to obtain a very clear history (see Urinary Symptoms).

Alimentary symptoms are occasionally of importance (e.g. a malignant ovarian tumour may first present with epigastric discomfort, nausea and anorexia) but usually bowel symptoms indicate a bowel problem.

Another frequent problem is vaginal discharge and clues as to its aetiology may be obtained from the history (see Vaginal Discharge).

Details of contraceptive methods are relevant in cases of secondary amenorrhoea, secondary subfertility, and pelvic inflammation and in patients requesting sterilisation.

Details of the past medical and surgical history, family and social history are obviously important.

GYNAECOLOGICAL EXAMINATION

You need to remember that the patient may well have either an undiagnosed concurrent, non-gynaecological disorder, or a local manifestation of a generalised disorder, so it is most important to conduct a full clinical examination, including urinalysis. Hypertension, diabetes, and breast lumps are not infrequently found in the gynaecological clinic.

The examination of the abdomen should *not* be confined to the lower abdomen, but should be thorough, checking for masses and any tenderness. Note any laparotomy or laparoscopy scars. It is most embarrassing for any patient, but particularly some older ladies, to be subjected to a pelvic examination, therefore adopt a technique which covers as much of the patient as possible. When you have completed the examination, cover the patient completely and reassure her, where possible, of normal findings.

Pelvic examination — as in all examinations — begins with inspection, noting any congenital abnormalities of the vulva or Bartholin's swellings. It is particularly important in vulval lesions to check for any inguinal lymphadenopathy. A vaginal speculum is carefully inserted with the patient in the dorsal or left lateral position. When a prolapse is present, you will have to use a Sims' speculum with the patient in the left lateral position. This allows access and assessment of the anterior vaginal wall. If you are attempting to elicit stress incontinence, the patient should have a full bladder. If a discharge is present, specimens may be obtained for bacteriological examination. The cervix may be inspected, and a smear taken for cytological assessment. Look for any local lesion or atrophic changes. Then, after ensuring that the patient has recently emptied her bladder, perform a bimanual examination which permits you to determine the size, shape, position, and mobility of the uterus, and the presence of any adnexal mass or inflammation. Some gynaecologists advocate bimanual examination before speculum examination, arguing that prior palpation will allow judgment of the correct size of speculum and thus reduce the chance of causing the patient discomfort. However, palpation before inspection may produce bleeding from surface lesions and obscure the field. One should, in any case, be able to judge the size of the introitus when inspecting the vulva.

In the event of a malignant disease you can determine the extent of spread. A rectal examination is mandatory.

After taking the history and performing an examination it should be possible to arrive at a provisional diagnosis (or *short* list of differential diagnoses). Appropriate special investigations may then be performed to confirm the diagnosis. Special investigations should not be requested blindly as a routine or as a substitute for a full history and examination.

GYNAECOLOGICAL EMERGENCIES

Emergencies presenting to the gynaecologist are varied, ranging from lesions of the vulva (Bartholin's abscesses or cysts, or vulval injuries), to vaginal haemorrhage and abdomino-pelvic pain. In practice, the common emergencies are those of *bleeding per vaginam* and *abdomino-pelvic pain* or both.

Most cases of urgent bleeding per vaginam are related to abortion (see p. 11). Occasionally menorrhagia or heavy irregular bleeding from a local lesion of the vulva, vagina or cervix may necessitate hospital admission but these cases are relatively rare.

Abdomino-pelvic pain is dealt with in greater detail in the subsequent chapters. However, the following information may be a useful guide to the beginner.

1. *Remember: the diagnosis of tubal pregnancy*
   The pain in this condition is varied in severity from an acute stabbing pain to intermittent colicky lower abdominal discomfort. It may be associated with shoulder-tip pain, syncopal attacks, or worsening on defaecation (all due to blood in the peritoneal cavity). A later feature may be bleeding per vaginam due to shedding of the decidua. The blood loss follows the pain, unlike abortion where bleeding is commonly the initial symptom. However, vaginal bleeding is not always present. Although menstrual disturbances are a common symptom, the absence of amenorrhoea does not exclude the diagnosis.
2. *Remember: general surgical conditions*
   Some surgical conditions may simulate gynaecological pathology: appendicitis and Crohn's disease may give right iliac fossa pain similar to that of an ovarian accident or tubal pregnancy; diverticular disease may similarly result in left

Table 1. Common gynaecological emergencies.

Condition	Symptoms					Signs			
	Amenorrhoea	Bleeding per vaginam	Pain	Vomiting	Pelvic mass	Cervical excitation Pelvic tenderness	Pulse Temperature	Blood pressure	Shock
Ectopic pregnancy	Commonly present but not reliable	Usually follows pain	Variable in severity, often sharp in lower abdomen and shouldertip	Not usual	Not common, restricted by tenderness	Usually very tender appendage +++	Tachycardia temperature slightly raised	Low when ruptures	Associated with tubal rupture
Ovarian accidents	Not often	No	Sudden onset Colicky leading to sharp stabbing	Yes	Yes, unless cyst ruptured	Pelvic tenderness ++	Tachycardia temperature raised	Normal	Not usual
Pelvic sepsis	Not usual	Occasional	Gradual onset Variable dull ache leading to peritonitis	Occasional	Variable restricted by tenderness	Marked cervical excitation and pelvic tenderness	Tachycardia and pyrexia	Normal	Only with septicaemic cases
Abortion	Yes	Yes	Dull ache, colicky with expulsion of tissue	Not usual	Uterine enlargement	Not usually tender unless post-abortal sepsis	Apyrexial pulse variable	Variable usually related to bleeding	Occasionally

iliac fossa pain.
3. *Remember: empty the bladder and exclude pregnancy*
   This is particularly important when a mass appears to be arising from the pelvis. Vigorous attempts to feel a mass when a tubal pregnancy is suspected are dangerous, especially at EUA. This may provoke tubal rupture and intra-peritoneal haemorrhage.
4. *Remember: vaginal examination*
   A pelvic examination is necessary in all cases with pelvic pain. Cervical excitation (pain on movement of the cervix) suggests irritation of the pelvic peritoneum which may result from an ectopic pregnancy, an ovarian cyst, sepsis or, more rarely, endometriosis.

   The state of the cervix, consistency, dilatation and the presence of blood in the os are valuable signs.
5. *Remember: rectal examination*
   This is particularly important when vaginal examination is not possible due to severe vaginismus or in a small child. It is also necessary to exclude surgical pathology.

Table 1 is a brief guide to the symptoms and signs of the more common gynaecological emergencies. It shows how there is a great overlap between conditions and the actual diagnosis may be difficult and may finally require laparoscopy or laparotomy. Since pelvic sepsis occurring in a normal pregnancy is rare, amenorrhoea associated with pelvic pain and tenderness is likely to indicate a tubal or ectopic pregnancy. A sudden onset of colicky pain and the presence of a mass more than 7.5 cm × 5 cm is suggestive of torsion of an ovarian cyst. Rarer conditions such as torsion of a pedunculated fibroid, acute bleeding or rupture of endometriotic cysts or torsion of a fallopian tube may simulate the commoner gynaecological emergencies. The presence of an acute abdomen or pelvic mass in a patient over forty years must arouse suspicion of neoplasia, a complication of fibroids or ovarian pathology. This may therefore require extensive surgery, and these cases should not be attempted by junior gynaecologists, unless under supervision.

1. SPECIFIC CONDITIONS

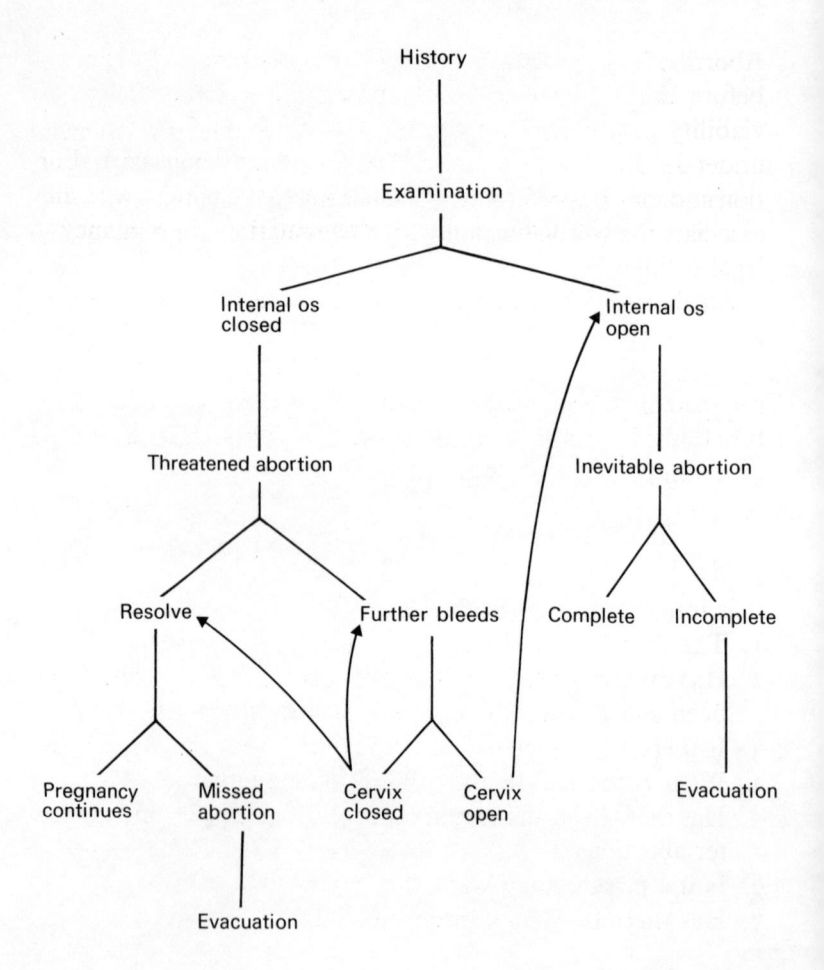

```
                        History
                           |
                      Examination
                      /           \
          Internal os              Internal os
          closed                   open
             |                        |
      Threatened abortion      Inevitable abortion
          /        \                /       \
      Resolve   Further bleeds   Complete  Incomplete
       /  \         |   \                      |
Pregnancy Missed  Cervix Cervix            Evacuation
continues abortion closed  open
            |
        Evacuation
```

(Cervix closed → Resolve / Further bleeds; Cervix open → Internal os open)

Abortion

Abortion is the discontinuation or termination of a pregnancy before the 28th week of gestation. The gestational age for viability may be revised to 20 or 24 weeks and is at present under debate. The term 'miscarriage' is synonymous with abortion and may be preferable when talking to the patient who may associate the word abortion with a termination of pregnancy — legal or illegal.

An abortion usually results in placental separation and bleeding per vaginam, followed by lower abdominal pain as the tissue is expelled from the uterus. Occasionally the fetus dies but is retained in utero; this is usually associated with continuing function of the trophoblastic tissue and is known as a 'missed abortion'.

History

It is important to ascertain:
1. The date of the patient's last menstrual period.
2. Has the patient had symptoms of early pregnancy and has it been confirmed clinically or by laboratory tests?
3. Is there any associated abdominal pain with the blood flow?
4. What is the nature and amount of the blood loss?
5. Has there been any loss of tissue (or liquor in second trimester abortions)?
6. Is it a planned and wanted pregnancy?
7. Has there been any 'interference'?

Examination

The patient's general condition should be assessed. Look for signs of shock and if necessary take appropriate resuscitative measures. Signs of infection (pyrexia and tachycardia) should be sought and you should examine the abdomen for evidence of uterine enlargement, masses, tenderness, and signs of peritonism, as ectopic pregnancy is one of the differential diagnoses. Then perform a speculum and bimanual examination to check whether the internal os is open and to confirm that the blood is coming through the cervix. The presence of an offensive discharge is strongly suggestive of infection. Note any pelvic tenderness and feel for the presence of an appendage mass which may be an ectopic pregnancy. Caution should be exercised in doing vaginal examinations on patients with a history of abortions, as the patient may attribute the subsequent loss of her pregnancy to the examination. However, it is a poor and likely a doomed pregnancy which cannot survive a gentle examination.

Management

Blood should be taken for estimation of the haemoglobin level and for 'group and save serum'. In cases where vaginal bleeding is heavy, cross-matched blood should be requested. The Rhesus factor should be determined in all cases and, if found to be negative, anti-D gammaglobulin should be given within 48 hours of abortion or evacuation.

Internal os closed

The commonest causes of first trimester abortions are associated with chromosomal abnormalities or faulty implantation, in which events abortion will usually occur irrespective of management.

The present management of threatened abortion tends to be bed rest whilst there is active bleeding, then mobilisation.

The authors consider that the use of progestogen injections

should be reserved only for cases of demonstrated progesterone deficiency.

Urinary immunological pregnancy tests detect the presence of hCG and, although a positive result usually indicates a viable pregnancy, it can also occur when the fetus has died but viable trophoblast remains. Ultrasonic scans are more reliable. If the bleeding resolves and the pregnancy continues there is no reason to believe that the pregnancy has been harmed by the bleed.

In *missed abortions* the bleeding settles but the uterus fails to grow. Objective parameters show a non-viable pregnancy. Although spontaneous evacuation eventually will occur, there is a risk of infection and hypofibrinogenaemia may develop after some four weeks. The uterus should therefore be evacuated — by dilatation and curettage or by suction, if under 12 weeks' size, or by extra-amniotic prostaglandins, if larger.

Internal os open

When the cervix opens and the products protrude into the canal, a diagnosis of inevitable abortion can be made. This will lead to uterine emptying, either complete or incomplete. The presence of remaining products in the uterus may result in haemorrhage or infection so that evacuation is necessary. Products in the cervical canal may lead to a degree of shock out of proportion to the amount of blood lost; this is known as 'cervical shock' and responds dramatically to the removal of the products. Products in the os may also cause persistent bleeding which usually stops quickly if the products are removed.

Haemorrhage should be controlled by 0.5 mg ergometrine intravenously, supported by an infusion of 10 units of oxytocin in 500 ml of 5% dextrose until the evacuation can be carried out. You should send all products evacuated from the uterus for histological examination to confirm the pregnancy and exclude trophoblastic disease. Curettings showing decidua but no chorionic villi are suggestive of an ectopic pregnancy.

Patients who have suffered an abortion are often upset and concerned about future pregnancies. As the most common cause of isolated early abortions is a non recurring fetal abnormality, the patients may be strongly reassured, pointing out that possibly 15–20% of conceptions end as spontaneous abortions. There is no medical reason to defer further conception and the couple may try for a further pregnancy whenever they are ready. You should advise the patient to report to her family practitioner as soon as she thinks she is pregnant.

Comment

Abortion is one of the commonest causes of maternal death and, together with its complications, constitutes a high percentage of gynaecological emergencies. Its importance in medical practice, not only to the gynaecologist but also the general practitioner, cannot be over-emphasised.

Shock associated with abortion must arouse suspicion of sepsis and 'criminal' interference. The latter is now fortunately less common since the introduction of the 1967 Abortion Act.

A diagnosis of 'abortion' before the eighth week of amenorrhoea may be spurious. There may be a pregnancy in the fallopian tube.

Some women suffer repeated abortions and, if a patient has had three confirmed successive abortions, she comes into a category known as 'recurrent or habitual aborters'. Several possible causative factors have been postulated and require investigating before the next pregnancy: these include maternal, uterine and chromosomal factors.

Maternal factors include chronic disorders such as renal disease, syphilis, diabetes mellitus, thyroid deficiency, rhesus iso-immunisation, folate deficiency, and progesterone deficiency. Whilst some of these factors are widely accepted, others are in question — particularly folate deficiency and progesterone deficiency. Vaginal wall smears taken during a pregnancy with a threatened abortion may show signs of progesterone deficiency, but it is difficult to prove that the deficiency is the cause of the bleeding and not merely another manifestation of an abnormal pregnancy.

Uterine factors are threefold. 1. Anatomical fusion defects may interfere with correct implantation — as may submucous fibroids. 2. Cervical incompetence is a well recognised cause of recurrent late abortion and, whilst it may occur spontaneously, it usually follows cervical damage either from laceration at a previous delivery or termination of pregnancy, or from excessive dilatation at termination, diagnostic curettage or as a 'cure' for spasmodic dysmenorrhoea. 3. Surgical damage includes cone biopsy or amputation at prolapse repair.

Chromosomal factors. Recent advances in cytogenetic techniques and wider availability of facilities has shown that, in a small number of recurrent aborters, subtle chromosomal factors are present.

Before these patients conceive again these factors should be looked for and investigations should include renal function, serological tests for syphilis, glucose tolerance, thyroid function, folate levels, Rhesus factor and antibody levels (if appropriate), hysterosalpingography in the luteal phase of the cycle to show any uterine anomaly or cervical problem, and genetic counselling. Any abnormal finding should be treated appropriately but, in the majority of cases, the cause is idiopathic.

These women are often, understandably, very anxious and require a sympathetic approach with ample reassurance. Even if no abnormality is found and no treatment is given, they have a 50% chance of carrying the next pregnancy to term. As these patients may be very demanding they often receive empirical treatments for which there is no definite indication; these may include folate supplements, progesterone injections, hCG injections, and Shirodkar suture. Whilst folate or hCG are apparently harmless, progesterone injections may cause masculinisation of female fetuses and inserting a suture may stimulate uterine activity and cause an abortion. Treatment should therefore be restricted to demonstrated abnormalities.

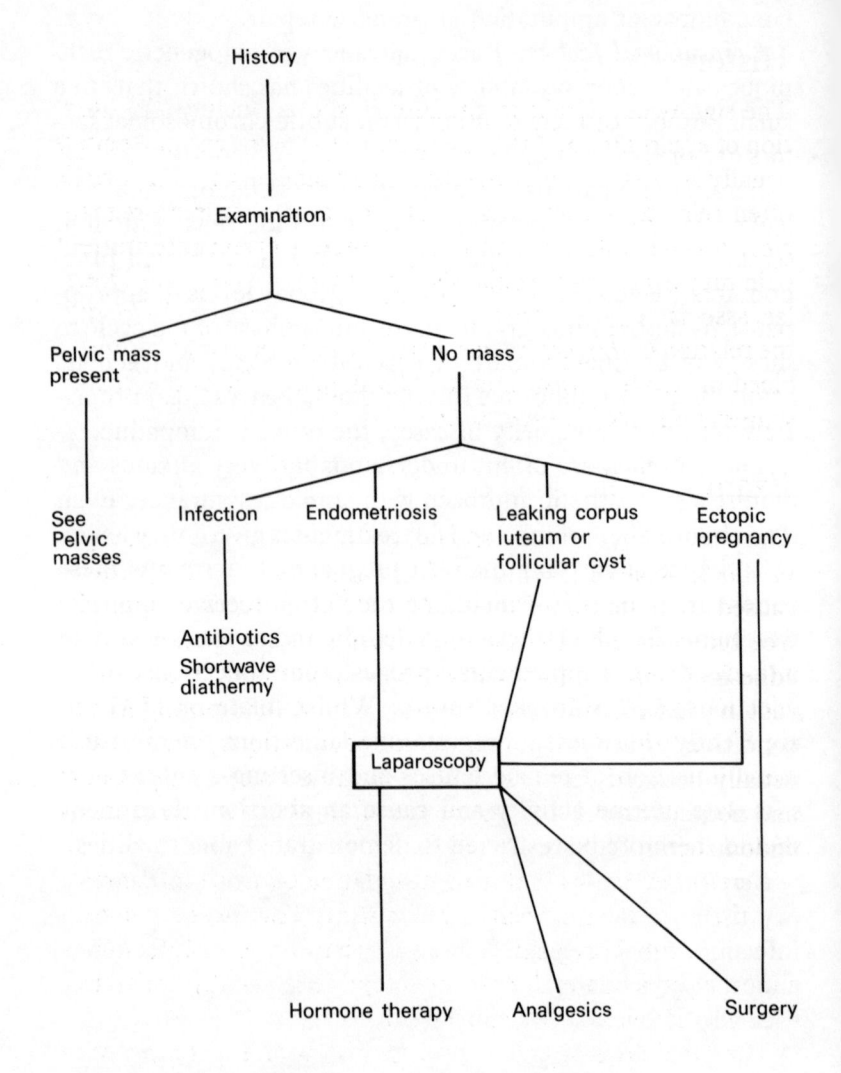

```
History
  │
  │
Examination
  │
  ├─────────────────────────────────┐
Pelvic mass                        No mass
present                              │
  │                    ┌────────┬────┴────────┬──────────────┐
  │                Infection  Endometriosis  Leaking corpus  Ectopic
See                     │                    luteum or       pregnancy
Pelvic                  │                    follicular cyst
masses              Antibiotics
                    Shortwave
                    diathermy
                                    │         │              │
                                    └──┬──────┴──────────────┘
                                   [Laparoscopy]
                              ┌────────┼────────┐
                         Hormone    Analgesics  Surgery
                         therapy
```

Pelvic Pain

History

The significant details in the history should include the duration of symptoms and the character of the pain (chronic pain is usually associated with infection or endometriosis; acute pain is often related to 'accidents' to ovarian cysts, ectopic pregnancies, leaking follicles and corpus luteum cysts; intermittent pain may occur with 'prolapsed ovaries' in the pouch of Douglas, associated with retroversion).(See Dyspareunia.) Secondly, the relation of the pain to periods (mid-cycle pain may be due to bleeding from an ovarian follicle, a period of amenorrhoea suggests an ectopic pregnancy).

Examination

The patient's general condition should be assessed, noting signs of shock, anaemia, shoulder tip pain when lying flat, (this is caused by irritation of the undersurface of the diaphragm by free blood in the peritoneum), fixation of the uterus (due to adhesions, either inflammatory or endometriotic), retroversion (not in itself a cause of pain but associated with some underlying condition, either inflammatory or endometriotic, when it will usually be fixed), and thickening of the uterosacral ligaments and nodules palpable in the pouch of Douglas (which suggests endometriotic deposits).

Cervical excitation is due to stimulation of *active* inflammatory tissue, reflecting pelvic peritonism. This may be due to infection, tubal pregnancy, or an ovarian accident. Infection is almost always bilateral, cysts or ectopics are usually unilateral. (See also Pelvic Masses and Dysmenorrhoea.)

The tubal distension may be palpable but, if tubal rupture or abortion has occurred, no mass will be felt. Pelvic tenderness and cervical excitation are more reliable signs of an ectopic pregnancy than the presence of a mass.

Management

There may be symptoms and signs of free blood in the peritoneum (e.g. syncope, shoulder tip pain, guarding, rebound tenderness), or pelvic haematocele. If there is any doubt and an ectopic pregnancy cannot be excluded, a *diagnostic laparoscopy* should be performed.

If the patient is clinically shocked, an urgent laparotomy is indicated. Any delay in an attempt to resuscitate the patient may result in death, the blood transfused being lost as fast as it can be given.

In a significant number of patients no abnormality can be found on examination but, in view of the patient's symptoms, laparoscopy is performed and, when it is, no abnormality whatsoever can be found. This condition, sometimes called the pelvic pain syndrome, is often difficult to treat. In common with dyspareunia and dysmenorrhoea, pelvic pain is a condition which is apparently influenced to a great extent by psychological factors and, in patients with emotional or social problems, many symptoms become magnified. A sympathetic discussion with the patient may help but often the symptoms are unchanged and it is not unknown for the patient to attend numerous gynaecologists. Eventually some end up having a hysterectomy but still have problems.

Comment

The laparoscope is a useful tool in the diagnosis of pelvic pain but the dangers and contra-indications to laparoscopy should not be overlooked (see p. 112).

A more rational approach to the treatment of salpingitis would be to culture the organisms from the fallopian tube, which may be achieved via the laparascope. The occurrence of the 'pelvic pain syndrome' should be remembered. Surgery should be avoided in the absence of visible pathology.

Low Back Pain

Less than 1% of cases of low back pain are due solely to a gynaecological cause. Most are due to 'wear and tear' on the bones, joints and ligaments — a price we pay for an upright, bipedal posture.

The usual *causes* of low back pain are: osteoarthritis of the intervertebral joints, sacroiliac joints, sacralisation of L5 vertebra, scoliosis, kyphosis, osteoporosis, sacro-iliac strain, and ligamentous or muscular strain associated with heavy work or obesity.

Uterine and vaginal prolapse do not cause backache but rather a dragging discomfort which is relieved by lying down. Pre-menstrual pelvic congestion, or that associated with pelvic inflammation or endometriosis, may exacerbate an existing problem, so that the patient refers the pain to menstruation. Pain associated with tumours is a rare and late feature. Bony metastases or tuberculosis of the spine are rare.

An X-ray of the lumbosacral spine and sacro-iliac joints is indicated; thereafter an orthopaedic opinion may be required.

Comment

One should *never* operate on a patient with a prolapse whose *sole* complaint is low back pain — she will not be cured and you will have a most unhappy patient.

A retroverted uterus is rarely the cause of symptoms (see Dyspareunia) unless it is associated with pathology such as endometriosis.

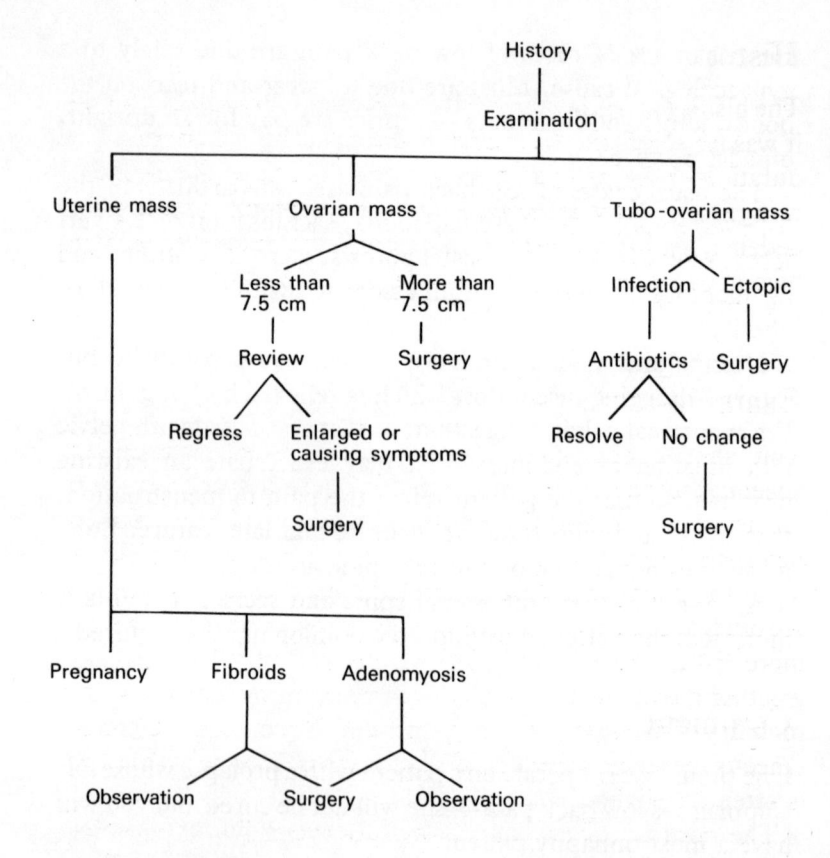

```
                              History
                                |
                           Examination
    _____|_____
    |                           |                           |
Uterine mass              Ovarian mass              Tubo-ovarian mass
    |                    _____|_____                _____|_____
    |                    |           |                |           |
    |              Less than    More than         Infection    Ectopic
    |               7.5 cm       7.5 cm              |           |
    |                 |            |              Antibiotics  Surgery
    |              Review       Surgery          ____|____
    |              __|__                         |       |
    |              |   |                      Resolve  No change
    |          Regress Enlarged or                       |
    |                  causing symptoms                Surgery
    |                      |
    |                   Surgery
    |
    |_____
    |              |                         |
Pregnancy      Fibroids                 Adenomyosis
                __|__                        |
                |   |                        |
          Observation Surgery          Observation
```

Pelvic Masses

History

The history should determine how the mass presented: whether it was an accidental finding or was producing symptoms. The duration of the symptoms may give a clue to its likelihood of malignancy. Note associated signs or symptoms such as pain, oedema, or breathlessness. Menstrual disturbances, such as menorrhagia, are more likely with a uterine mass.

Examination

You should perform a general examination, noting any anaemia, jaundice, lymphadenopathy, or any other evidence of metastases. It is essential that the patient empties her bladder before the examination. The shape, size, regularity, and mobility of the mass should be determined: smaller ovarian masses are often mobile and prone to torsion, whereas larger masses are more liable to feel fixed. It may be difficult to distinguish whether the mass is uterine or ovarian; one way is to assess the mobility of the mass with movement of the cervix since simultaneous movement suggests a uterine mass. However this sign is often unreliable.

The position of the mass is usually unhelpful when it has attained the size greater than a twelve week pregnancy. Both uterine and ovarian tumours tend to be centrally located, giving central dullness to percussion and resonance in the flanks, unless there is associated ascites.

Uterine mass

Fibromyomata or *fibroids* are typically multiple and cause an irregular mass. They are usually painless, unless they are undergoing degeneration or sarcomatous change, and their commonest presenting symptom is menorrhagia. If they are asymptomatic and less than the size of a ten week pregnancy, it is permissable to keep the patient under observation. When larger or causing symptoms, then surgery may be indicated — either myomectomy or hysterectomy. If the patient wishes to retain her fertility or finds hysterectomy unacceptable for cultural reasons, then myomectomy is performed. If the patient has completed her family then total hysterectomy is the treatment of choice.

Adenomyosis or *internal endometriosis* causes regular uterine enlargement (usually no larger than the size of a twelve week pregnancy) which is often tender. It responds poorly to hormone therapy (unlike external endometriosis) and, if troublesome, may require total hysterectomy. It may also be difficult to distinguish clinically between adenomyosis and a solitary fibroid.

Ovarian masses

These may be palpable vaginally or, if greater than the size of a twelve week pregnancy, in the abdomen, when they may occupy a central position. Smaller masses or 'cysts' (less than 7.5 cm) are usually palpable in the lateral fornix. They may be due to follicular or luteal cysts (exaggerated physiological responses) which may regress spontaneously, so it may be permissible to review the patient in four weeks.

Surgery is indicated for all ovarian tumours over 7.5 cm diameter (whether they are symptomatic or not) because of the risk of complications, such as torsion or haemorrhage, and the possibility of malignant change. Most benign cysts can be 'shelled' out of the ovarian tissue (cystectomy).

The presence of ascites, bilateral tumours, seedling deposits in the omentum and peritoneum, or solid areas in a cyst are *suggestive* of malignancy. However, ascites may occur in some benign conditions such as fibroma of the ovary; therefore the presence of ascites should not, on its own, be regarded as a contra-indication to surgery.

The presence of ovarian enlargements, of *any* size, in post-menopausal patients requires laparotomy.

Tubo-ovarian masses

The treatment of tubo-ovarian masses is similar to that of pelvic infection or inflammatory disease. If the patient does not respond to conservative management, or develops a pelvic abscess, then surgery may be necessary.

The possibility that the mass may be an ectopic pregnancy should always be considered, although these are usually associated with pelvic tenderness and may have a history of menstrual disturbance.

Comment

You should inspect both ovaries closely before beginning ovarian surgery. Where possible, in the young patient with a benign-looking lesion, *conservation* of ovarian tissue is the key word. However, ovarian tumours occurring in patients over 40 years should be regarded with the highest suspicion of malignancy: there is no place in these cases for ovarian cystectomy. Indeed, the policy when in doubt of the nature of an ovarian lesion, should be to take it *all* out.

The best results for primary ovarian carcinoma are obtained by removal of as much of the tumour as possible, supported by chemotherapy.

There is no question that early diagnosis is the most important factor in the prognosis. The active management of all masses over 7.5 cm cannot be over-emphasised.

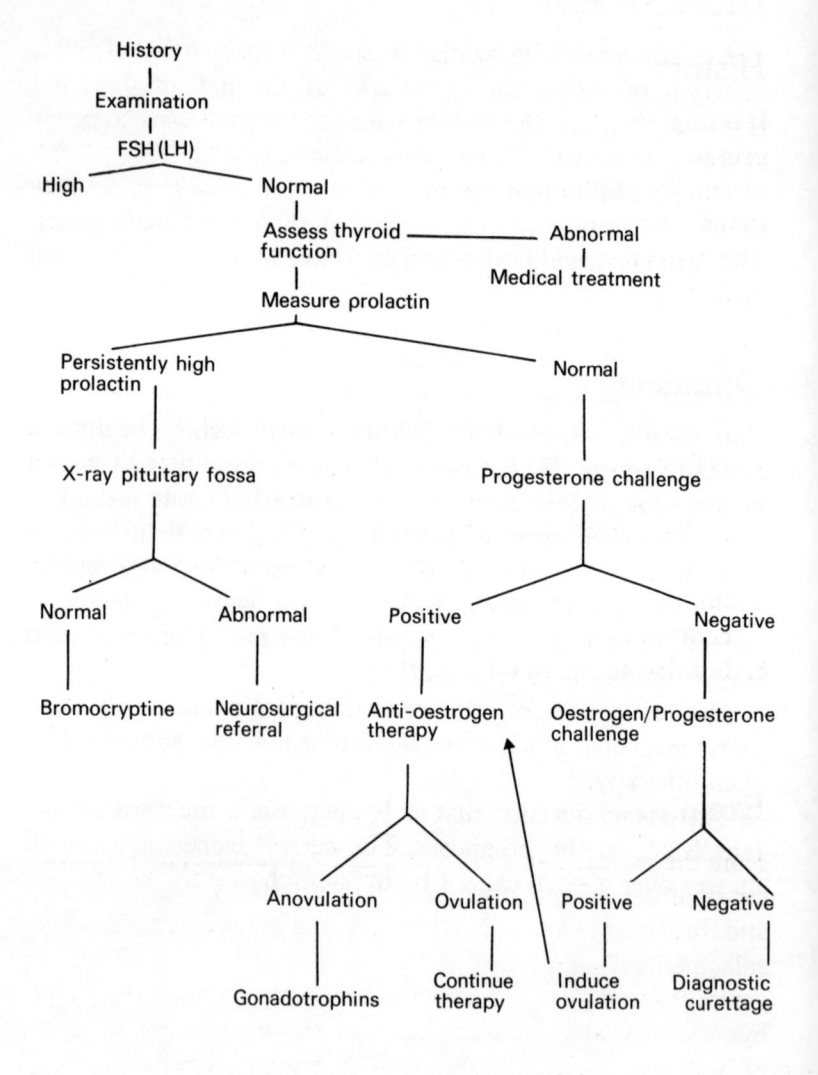

```
                    History
                       |
                　 Examination
                       |
                    FSH (LH)
              ┌────────┴────────┐
            High              Normal
                                |
                         Assess thyroid ──────── Abnormal
                           function                 |
                                |              Medical treatment
                         Measure prolactin
              ┌─────────────────┴─────────────────┐
      Persistently high                         Normal
         prolactin                                |
              |                           Progesterone challenge
      X-ray pituitary fossa                ┌──────┴──────┐
         ┌────┴────┐                    Positive      Negative
      Normal    Abnormal                   |              |
         |         |                  Anti-oestrogen   Oestrogen/Progesterone
   Bromocryptine  Neurosurgical         therapy          challenge
                    referral         ┌─────┴─────┐    ┌─────┴─────┐
                                 Anovulation  Ovulation Positive  Negative
                                     |           |        |          |
                               Gonadotrophins Continue  Induce   Diagnostic
                                              therapy  ovulation curettage
```

Amenorrhoea

History

It is important for you to establish whether the amenorrhoea is primary (where menstruation has never previously occurred) or secondary, and, if primary, to exclude congenital and chromosomal anomalies.
The history should determine the following:
1. Is there any possibility of pregnancy, as this is the commonest cause of secondary amenorrhoea?
2. Is there any recent weight loss which may reflect systemic disease, such as tuberculosis, anorexia nervosa, malabsorption syndrome, diabetes mellitus, or neoplasia?
3. Is there any psychological upset such as leaving home, marital strife, changing jobs, or taking exams?
4. Is there any family history of tuberculosis or diabetes?
5. Is the patient taking any drugs which may suppress ovulation or raise the level of prolactin in the blood (e.g. oral contraceptives, phenothiazines, metoclopramide)?
6. Is there any galactorrhoea?

Examination

Note the patient's general health and appearance; pay particular attention to the secondary sexual characteristics (body hair and breast development), stature, breasts (for evidence of galactorrhoea), and signs of thyroid dysfunction. The external genitalia should be examined closely for any evidence of clitoral hypertrophy, absence of vagina, 'imperforate hymen', or signs of oestrogen deficiency. In cases of primary amenorrhoea, a gentle bimanual examination should determine the presence or absence of a uterus; if the patient is a virgin this may be determined by rectal examination.

Follicle stimulating hormone (FSH)

FSH levels give more information than those of luteinising hormone (LH) as there is a big overlap between normal and abnormal values for LH but very little overlap with FSH. However, a disproportionately raised LH level may be found in cases of polycystic ovary syndrome. FSH levels around five times normal values may be found in *ovarian failure*. Fertility cannot be restored but symptoms of hormone deprivation can be treated by hormone replacement therapy (HRT).

Hypothyroidism

Hypothyroidism may be a cause of amenorrhoea in its own right or it may cause hyperprolactinaemia which, in turn, may be the cause of amenorrhoea. Hypothyroidism should be treated adequately and the menstrual situation reviewed when the patient is euthyroid.

Hyperprolactinaemia

This can be caused by pituitary adenomata before they are large enough to produce radiological changes of the pituitary fossa, therefore X-rays should be repeated at yearly intervals. Tomography may be helpful. The patient's visual fields and optic fundi should also be checked regularly, if necessary by an ophthalmologist. Other causes of raised prolactin levels include phenothiazines, tricyclic antidepressants, methyl dopa, metoclopramide, and haloperidol. Galactorrhoea is present in less than a third of cases.

Bromocryptine. In the absence of detectable abnormality the patient can be reassured. Unless she particularly desires to menstruate or conceive, there is no need to induce ovulation but if this is necessary, use bromocryptine. Dosage starts at 2.5 mg daily for the first week, increasing by 2.5 mg daily at weekly intervals to an optimum dose of 7.5 mg daily. Treatment is discontinued when pregnancy occurs. Patients often experience nausea for the first 24-48 hours after each dosage increase; this usually passes off so it is important to warn patients in order that they will continue therapy. In addition, alcohol may react with bromocryptine to produce troublesome nausea. Restricted X-ray studies should be repeated at yearly intervals, as should the test of visual fields and optic fundi.

Progesterone challenge

Progesterone will act on an oestrogen-primed endometrium. A five day course of a progestogen (e.g. norethisterone 5 mg b.d. or t.d.s.) should be followed by a withdrawal bleed within 3-4 days of stopping therapy if the oestrogen levels are satisfactory. This is a sensitive test of endogenous oestrogen secretion.

If the progesterone challenge is *negative* this may reflect either inadequate oestrogen levels or endometrial disease. You can differentiate between these by giving a combined oestrogen and progesterone preparation and observing a withdrawal bleed. A useful regime is a one month course of a combined oral contraceptive. If no bleed occurs, a curettage should be performed to exclude tuberculosis or intra-uterine adhesions (Asherman's syndrome) in which there is destruction of the endometrium either by infection or following over-vigorous curettage. This leads to the formation of intra-uterine adhesions which obliterate the cavity. Sometimes these adhesions may be broken down and their re-formation lessened by leaving an intra-uterine contraceptive device *in situ*. In a few cases, pregnancy may occur and there will then be a risk of placenta accreta.

A *positive* progesterone challenge confirms a satisfactory endogenous oestrogen level and suggests anovulation as a cause for the amenorrhoea. An anti-oestrogen (such as clomiphene 50 mg daily for five days or tamoxifen 20 mg daily for five days), should lower circulating oestrogen levels; this will cause a rise in FSH secretion which in turn produces follicular maturation.

If ovulation occurs, a uterine bleed will occur approximately three weeks after the therapy. If ovulation does not occur, the dose can be increased up to three times above the first dosage but, if this still does not work, exogenous gonadotrophin therapy may be required.

For the detection of ovulation see Subfertility — Female.

Comment

The problem of post-pill amenorrhoea could be minimised by not prescribing the combined contraceptive pill to patients with a history of oligomenorrhoea, delayed menarche, or episodes of amenorrhoea.

It is important to recognise that amenorrhoea may be a symptom of systemic disease or psychological upset. This symptom should serve as a reminder that gynaecology is more than a surgical speciality of the female reproductive tract.

Having reassured the patient that she is normal, it is not necessary to continue therapy unless she particularly desires to menstruate or wishes to conceive.

Post-Menopausal Bleeding

Although the most common causes of post-menopausal bleeding (PMB) are exogenous oestrogen therapy and atrophic vaginitis due to oestrogen deficiency, all cases must be regarded as being due to malignancy until proven otherwise.

History
1. Was the patient receiving oestrogen therapy?
2. Was the bleeding *per vaginam*? It may be rectal or urethral.
3. Was the blood loss fresh or altered blood, and was it associated with a vaginal discharge?
4. Was there any post-coital bleeding?
5. Was there any associated pain?

Examination
This should determine the presence of local lesions of the vulva, vagina and cervix. A cervical smear should be taken and any bleeding from the cervix noted. Smears may also be taken from lesions in other sites (see Cytology). The size, shape and mobility of the uterus should be determined by bimanual examination. The appendages must be checked for swelling and tenderness. If the site of the bleeding is in doubt, a rectal examination should be performed as well as urine checked for haematuria.

Management
A diagnostic curettage is mandatory. A recurrent episode of bleeding following a negative curettage demands close attention. Rare causes of PMB include oestrogen-secreting ovarian

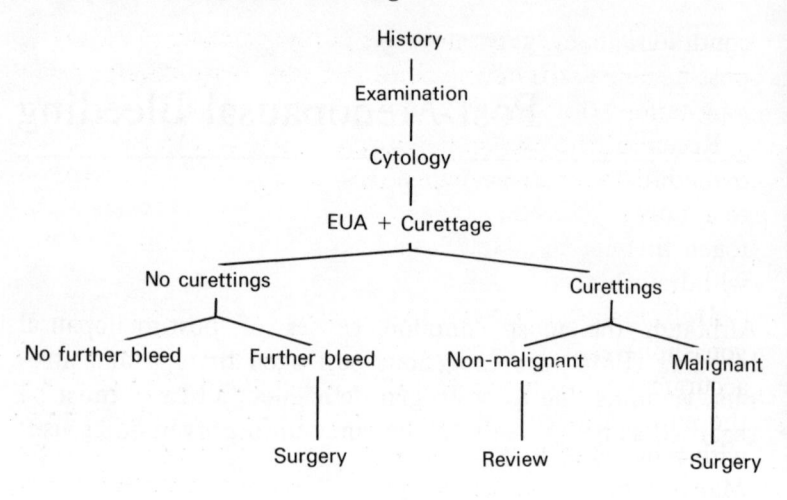

```
                    History
                       |
                  Examination
                       |
                   Cytology
                       |
                EUA + Curettage
              ┌────────┴────────┐
         No curettings      Curettings
          ┌────┴────┐       ┌────┴────┐
    No further   Further  Non-malignant  Malignant
      bleed      bleed         |            |
                   |         Review      Surgery
                Surgery
```

tumours, such as granulosa cell tumours, or carcinoma of the fallopian tube.

Post-menopausal uteri should not have any curettings, so even non-malignant endometrium warrants further follow-up. Occasionally, post-menopausal uteri may have endometrium showing hyperplasia. There are different histological patterns of hyperplasia from the cystic pattern, which are often associated with oestrogen administration and are usually regarded as ranging from benign to adenomatous. The latter often shows atypical features and is widely regarded as a pre-malignant condition.

If adenomatous hyperplasia is present, hysterectomy should be considered — especially if the histological appearances are atypical. The position is less clear with cystic hyperplasia: if exogenous oestrogens have been prescribed for menopausal symptoms, the hyperplasia should regress when the treatment is stopped and this may be confirmed by subsequent vacuum aspiration or curettage. If no exogenous oestrogens have been given, you should bear in mind the possibility of an oestrogen-secreting tumour. In obese patients the adipose tissue converts circulating adrenal sex steroids to active oestrogenic substances and this may be the cause of the hyperplasia. Although there is no firm evidence that cystic hyperplasia is a pre-malignant condition, many gynaecologists advise hysterectomy in the post-menopausal woman. If this is not performed, careful long-term follow-up is essential.

Recently progestogen therapy has become more widely used to modify the oestrogen-stimulated endometrium, converting it to a 'normal' secretory type of endometrium. Cyclical progestogen therapy (see Hormone Therapy) will permit a regular withdrawal bleed.

Malignant curettings are usually pale, bulky and friable, but you should await the results of histological examination for accurate diagnosis. The usual treatment of adenocarcinoma of the endometrium is surgical: total abdominal hysterectomy with removal of both tubes and ovaries, and a cuff of vagina. Many gynaecologists employ pre or post-operative radiotherapy. The tumour, particularly the well differentiated adenocarcinoma, may respond to progestogen therapy and this may be used in conjunction with surgery, for those patients unfit for surgery, or for recurrences.

The prognosis for carcinoma of the endometrium is usually good if an early diagnosis is made, but all patients should be followed-up indefinitely.

Comment

The presence of atrophic vaginitis or the history of exogenous oestrogen therapy does *not* exclude the diagnosis of carcinoma of the endometrium.

A curettage or endometrial biopsy must be performed in all cases, the method depending on the patient's fitness for anaesthesia. At the same time as the curettage, the bladder should be catheterised to facilitate the bimanual examination and check for haematuria.

If no 'cause' is found for the bleeding or if there is haematuria, cystoscopy should be performed to exclude a bladder lesion and a sigmoidoscopy to exclude a rectal lesion.

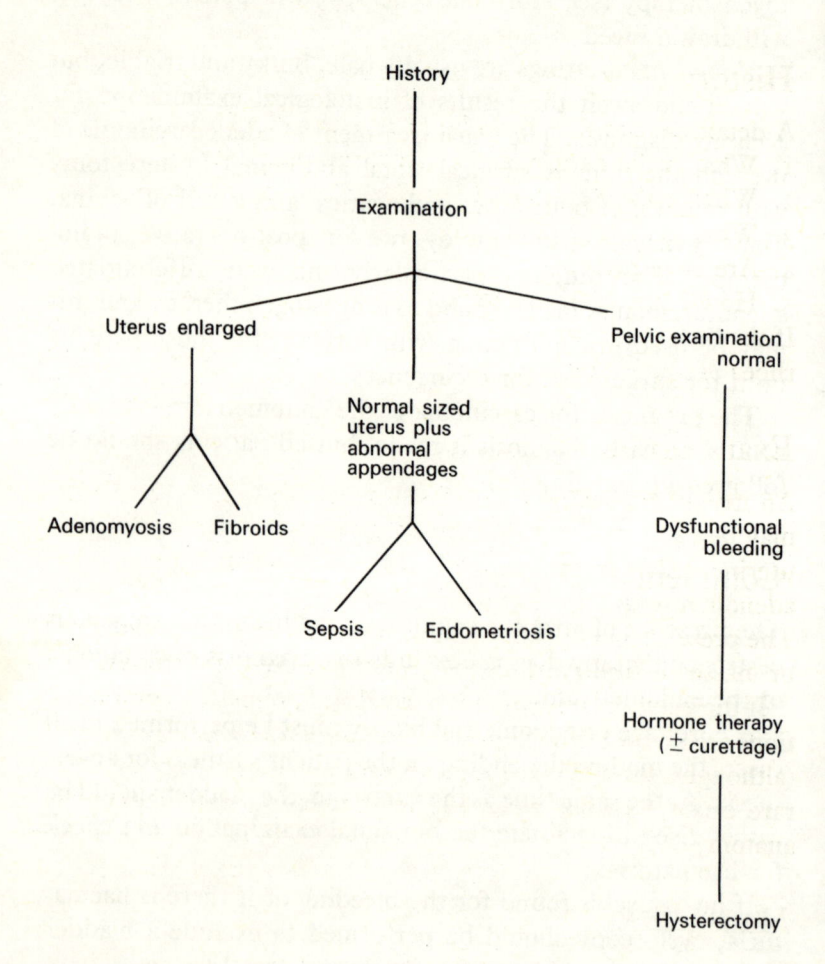

```
History
  │
Examination
  ├─────────────────┬─────────────────────┐
Uterus enlarged    Normal sized          Pelvic examination
  │                uterus plus            normal
  │                abnormal                  │
  │                appendages                │
  ├──────┐           ├──────┐                │
Adenomyosis Fibroids Sepsis Endometriosis    │
                                        Dysfunctional
                                         bleeding
                                             │
                                        Hormone therapy
                                        (± curettage)
                                             │
                                        Hysterectomy
```

Heavy or Irregular Menstruation

History
A detailed history is essential to ascertain the following:
1. What is the nature of the menstrual problem?
2. What is the duration of symptoms and of the flow?
3. What is the cycle frequency?
4. Are clots present?
5. How many pads or tampons are used per period?

If the bleeding is irregular or following an episode of amenorrhoea *pregnancy* must be excluded.

Examination
An irregularly *enlarged uterus* is usually due to fibroids which may be dealt with by myomectomy or hysterectomy. Regular uterine enlargement may be due to a solitary fibroid or adenomyosis and is dealt with in the section on Pelvic Masses. The presence of appendage thickening, tenderness, nodularity or masses is dealt with in the section on Dysmenorrhoea.

If the pelvic examination is normal and pregnancy complications are excluded, a diagnosis of *dysfunctional bleeding* is made (although a submucous fibroid or intra-uterine polyp could be a rare cause). This is a disorder of physiology rather than of anatomy.

Management
The most common cause of dysfunctional bleeding is hormone imbalance, which can be corrected by hormone therapy: either progestogens, oestrogen–progestogen combinations or, if found to be anovular in origin, an anti-oestrogen (e.g.

clomiphene). A common 'cause' of such hormonal imbalance appears to be related to psychological stresses such as marital disharmony, emotional upset, or sudden change of environment. The mechanism of this relationship is not clear.

In young patients, as in cases of dysmenorrhoea, curettage should be avoided if possible as the cervical dilatation may lead to an incompetent cervix.

Cyclical oestrogen-progestogen combinations are often an effective treatment, particularly when contraception is required. In cases where oestrogens are contra-indicated (e.g. hypertension, history of thrombo-embolism, etc.), cyclical progestogens may be employed (see Hormone Therapy). If these measures are ineffective, the anti-gonadotrophin, danazol, may be useful although the patient should be warned of possible amenorrhoea. Prolonged episodes of heavy bleeding can be arrested by using progestogens. Irregular bleeding and intermenstrual bleeding may also follow the use of depot progestogen injections for contraception or from 'breakthrough' bleeding on a low-dose contraceptive pill.

In some peri-menopausal patients, histological examination of the curettings may show hyperplasia. The significance of hyperplasia is much debated but, in general, there are two main types: *cystic hyperplasia* which is often associated with oestrogen stimulation unmodified by progesterone. There is no real evidence to suggest it is pre-malignant. Cyclical progestogen therapy is usually successful. These patients should be followed-up with vacuum aspirations or curettages and observed through the menopause. If any atypical factors develop, hysterectomy is advocated. *Adenomatous hyperplasia*, often with atypical histological features, is regarded by many gynaecologists and pathologists as a pre-malignant condition and total hysterectomy is usually advised. If this is not performed careful follow-up is mandatory with repeated endometrial biopsy by either vacuum aspiration or curettage.

Total hysterectomy should be reserved for those cases which fail to respond to conservative hormonal treatment or develop glandular atypia. There is very little place for an X-ray menopause.

Comment

Heavy blood loss at menstruation may be a difficult symptom to assess because of individual variation in the normal menstrual flow. The measure of loss by tampon or towel is rather inaccurate and, in part, reflects personal hygiene and fastidiousness —although a twofold increase in usage for a particular patient *is* significant. Such a heavy loss cannot be controlled by tampons alone. The passage of blood clot is related to heavy losses and arises when the blood flow overcomes the usual fibrinolytic mechanism present in the uterus. Clots greater than 2.5 cm in diameter are significant.

The question of post-sterilisation menorrhagia remains undecided; cause or coincidence? However, in patients requesting sterilisation with pre-existing menstrual problems, hysterectomy as a primary procedure may well be the treatment of choice.

Curettage has little therapeutic value but may be useful in the diagnosis of the pre-menopausal patient who may subsequently proceed to a carefully observed menopause.

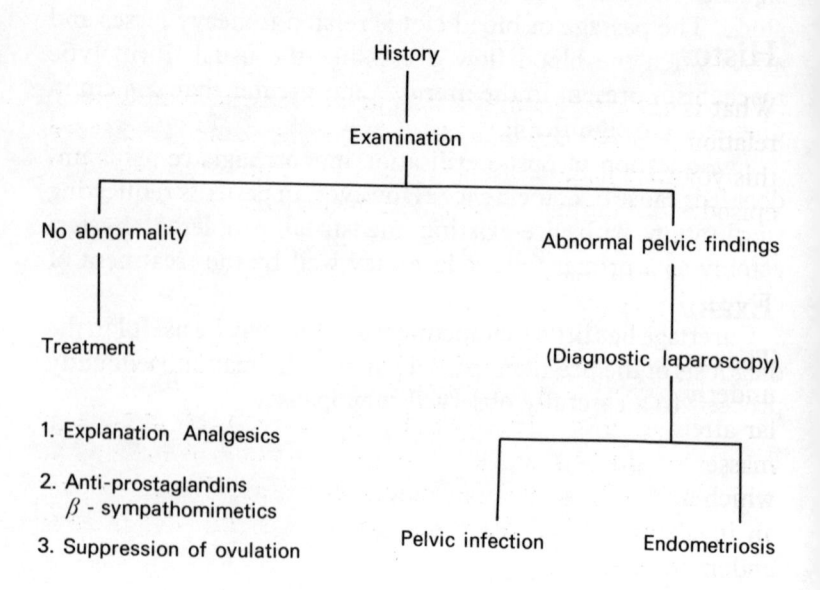

```
                    History
                       |
                  Examination
          _____|_____
         |                           |
   No abnormality            Abnormal pelvic findings
         |                           |
     Treatment              (Diagnostic laparoscopy)
                             _____|_____
                            |                 |
1. Explanation Analgesics

2. Anti-prostaglandins
   β - sympathomimetics

3. Suppression of ovulation
                        Pelvic infection   Endometriosis
```

Dysmenorrhoea

History

What is the site, nature, duration and time of pain onset in relation to menstrual flow? How bad is the pain? (To discover this you may need to ask about absence from work or school, episodes of fainting, or failure of analgesics).

Examination

The examination is important to determine whether there is any underlying pathology causing the dysmenorrhoea. Pay particular attention to the presence of pelvic tenderness, appendage masses or thickening, or a fixed retroversion of the uterus, which may reflect pelvic inflammatory disease. Laparoscopy is an invaluable aid in diagnosis, particularly in cases of early endometriosis.

Management

The underlying cause for the dysmenorrhoea should be treated appropriately. The three common types of dysmenorrhoea are, firstly, *spasmodic* — this occurs typically in women of 16–25 years, and only in ovulatory cycles (thus the first year or more after the menarche may not be painful). The pain starts before the menstrual loss and passes off usually within twelve hours. The cause is ill-understood, although it is more common in anxious, introspective girls who are relatively ignorant of menstrual physiology. Secondly, *congestive* — this is often secondary to pelvic infection. The pain gradually increases from about a week before the period as the pelvic organs become congested, and usually eases as the menstrual flow commences and the congestion lessens. These patients often have deep dyspareunia (see p. 41). This type of dysmenorrhoea often responds to the treatment of the underlying pelvic inflammation. Thirdly, *endometriosis* — the pain is similar to that of pelvic congestion except that it continues and may worsen with the flow as the ectopic endometrium sheds blood.

In some cases of spasmodic dysmenorrhoea explanation of menstruation and reassurance, together with *mild* analgesics, will help. However, several girls have severe discomfort and they may be helped by anti-prostaglandin agents (e.g. mefanamic acid, indomethacin) or β-sympathomimetic agents (e.g. orciprenaline, salbutamol). If these measures are ineffective, or if contraception is also required, ovulation suppression using a combined oestrogen-progesterone pill will alleviate symptoms in almost all patients.

Pelvic infection may be difficult to treat as it is not usually possible to obtain suitable specimens for culturing the causative organism; treatment must therefore be 'blind'. Usual antibiotic treatment includes a broad spectrum agent such as ampicillin or cotrimoxazole. There is some evidence to suggest that anaerobic organisms are a common cause and these respond to metronadizole. Some authorities have suggested that bacteroides are also a common cause and these may respond to agents such as lincomycin or clindamycin (see Drug Therapy).

Treatment needs to be more prolonged than is usual for other infections in view of the chronic nature of the problem. In order to further increase the blood flow in the area, many gynaecologists recommend a course of short wave diathermy to the pelvis. Different regimes are in use, a common one being twice weekly treatments of 20–30 minutes for six weeks. The resulting hyperaemia may or may not influence the course of the disease but the effects on the patient can be dramatic. Many complain of a temporary worsening of the pain after each treatment and, unless advised of this possibility in advance, may discontinue the treatment. If suitably advised beforehand the discomfort may prove to be of positive psychological benefit (see also Pelvic Pain and Pelvic Masses).

Endometriosis often causes ovarian enlargement due to bleeding into deposits on the ovary producing chocolate cysts. There may also be deposits on the uterosacral ligaments. However, there is little relation between the size of the deposits and the pain experienced. If endometriosis is suspected, a laparoscopy should be performed to confirm its presence and extent. In a small number of cases, surgery may be required but hormone therapy is the treatment of choice, and may include: danazol, progesterone, oestrogen-progesterone combinations, or dydrogesterone. (For further details see Hormone Therapy.)

Comment

There is very little value in cervical dilatation in cases of dysmenorrhoea except when *all* other methods have failed. Excessive dilatation of the cervix (especially beyond 10mm) may render it incompetent in subsequent pregnancies.

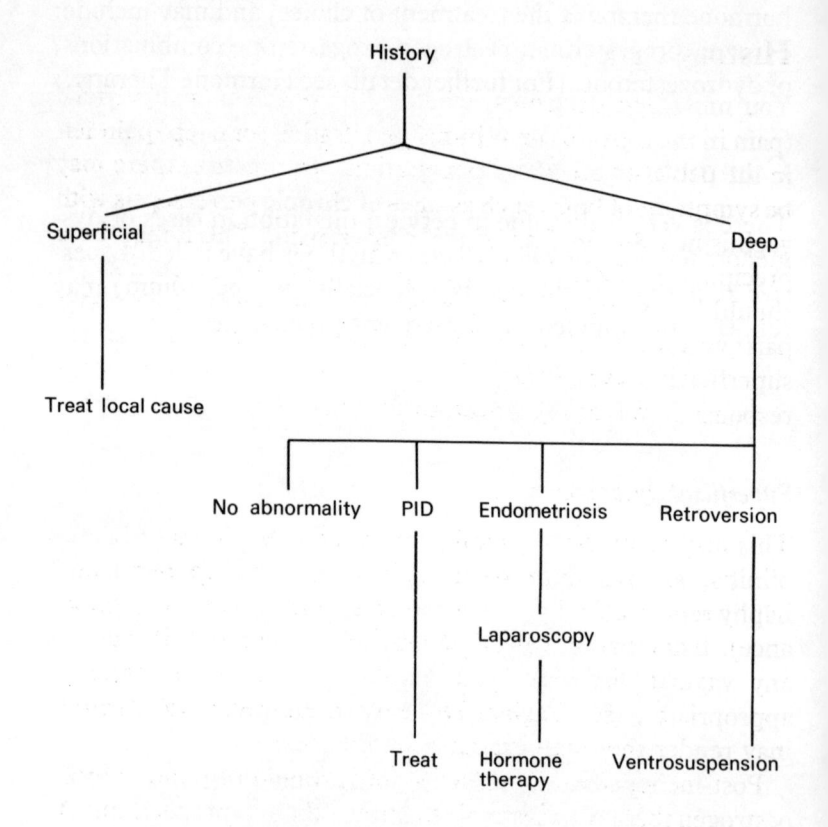

```
                          History
                         /      \
                  Superficial   Deep
                       |          |
              Treat local cause   |
                                  |
        ┌──────────┬──────────┬──────────┐
   No abnormality  PID   Endometriosis  Retroversion
                    |         |              |
                    |    Laparoscopy         |
                    |         |              |
                  Treat   Hormone      Ventrosuspension
                          therapy
```

Dyspareunia

History

You must first determine whether the problem is superficial (pain in the introitus or at initial penetration) or deep (pain felt in the pelvis on advanced penetration). In practice, there may be symptoms of both, such as cases of chronic pelvis sepsis with vaginismus due to fear of the deeper pain. There may be a precipitating factor, e.g. post-partum or post-operation. It should be remembered that psychological factors often play a part: vaginismus of psychological origin is a common cause for superficial dyspareunia. Psychological factors are often responsible for cases of deep dyspareunia (see Pelvic Pain).

Superficial dyspareunia

This may result from a local problem, e.g. vaginitis or Bartholinitis, an over-enthusiastic episiotomy or colpoperineorrhaphy repair, atrophy, or psychological factors (fear and ignorance). Examination will reveal any local cause and, if there is any vaginal discharge, you should investigate and treat it appropriately (see Vaginal Discharge). However, vaginismus may render thorough examination difficult.

Post-menopausal, atrophic vaginitis should respond to local oestrogen therapy or systemic therapy if the symptoms recur. A tender scar or excessive closure at repair of an episiotomy or prolapse may warrant surgical correction or the use of dilators. Psychological causes may respond to psychosexual counselling.

Deep dyspareunia

This is usually related to pathology, such as chronic pelvic inflammatory disease or endometriosis (see Dysmenorrhoea and Pelvic Pain), but you should bear in mind the effects of psychological factors.

A retroverted uterus carries the ovaries to the pouch of Douglas, where they may be reached on intercourse, causing a typical pain which settles soon after ceasing contact. The pain may radiate to the perineum and to the inner aspect of the thigh. It may be reproduced on bimanual examination when the ovary is palpated. If the uterus is mobile, some gynaecologists choose to correct the retroversion and insert a Hodge pessary to maintain anteversion. This is useful as a test to determine whether operation will provide a definitive cure; however, it is only a temporary measure and, if successful, a ventrosuspension should be offered. If there is a fixed retroversion, the underlying cause must be determined and treated appropriately (see also Dysmenorrhoea).

Comment

A sympathetic, reassuring approach is essential in establishing the patient's confidence. In some cases it is possible to demonstrate to the patient that there are no mechanical problems with intercourse by performing a gentle bimanual examination.

Pruritus Vulvae

History

1. Is the pruritus generalised or localised to the vulva?
2. Is the itch solely vulval or is there an anal irritation?
3. Is there an associated vaginal discharge?
4. Has the patient any dyspareunia?
5. Is the patient taking any drugs or using local applications such as deodorant sprays, or applying any ointments or antiseptic creams?
6. Is there likely to be any dietary deficiency or vitamin lack?
7. Is there a past history of diabetes mellitus, intestinal resection, malabsorption, vitamin B_{12} deficiency, blood dyscrasia or psoriasis?
8. Is there a psychiatric history?

Examination

A general examination is mandatory to exclude lymphadenopathy, splenomegaly, jaundice, anaemia, scabies, fungal infections, stomatitis, and glossitis. You should also perform a local examination to check for vaginal discharge, atrophy, or trophic changes in the vulva. Note any signs of excoriation, ulceration or condylomata, and examine urine for protein and glucose.

Generalised pruritus

This may be caused by lymphomata (Hodgkin's disease), leukaemia, uraemia, jaundice, deficiency states (vitamin B_{12}, B_2, A and iron), and achlorhydria. To detect these causes you need to make special investigations which may include: urea,

Pruritus Vulvae

```
                        History
                           |
                       Examination
                      /            \
           Generalised              Localised
            pruritus                 pruritus
               |                    /        \
           Specific           Discharge    No discharge
        investigations         present       present
                                  |
                             Specific treatment
                             /            \
                      Pruritus          Pruritus
                      resolves          persists
                                              |
                                   /                    \
                         No visible changes        Visible changes
                                  |                       |
                              Specific              Specific
                           investigations        investigations
                           /          \                 |
                       Normal       Abnormal        Histology
                          |            |             /      \
                     General and    Specific     Benign    Premalignant
                     local measures therapy         |      or malignant
                                                General       |
                                                and local   Surgery
                                                measures
```

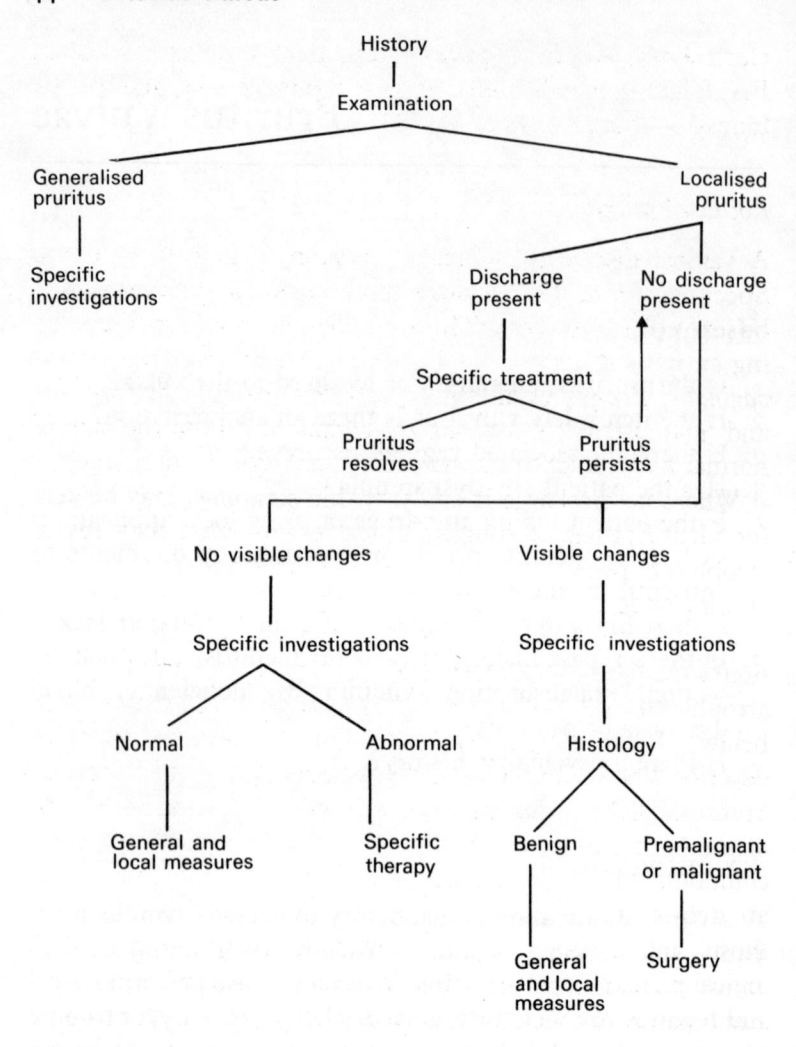

electrolytes, liver function tests, full blood count (iron, vitamin B_{12}, folate — if indicated), glucose tolerance test, and a node biopsy — if appropriate.

Localised pruritus

A vaginal discharge is present in more than 50% of cases. Specimens from the discharge (both pipette and swab) should be sent to the laboratory. The more common organisms producing an itchy discharge are *Candida albicans* and *Trichomonas vaginalis*. Pre-pubertally and post-menopausally opportunist and 'non-specific' infections are common, due to the lack of normal body defence mechanisms (see Vaginal Discharge).

Where no discharge is evident, skin scrapings may be sent for identification of fungi. Clinical examination may reveal atrophy, hypoplastic or hyperkeratotic changes, or there may be no visible change at all.

Visible changes merit cytological and histological examination: a small lesion may be usefully 'treated' by excision biopsy; atrophic changes may be treated by local oestrogen therapy (see below). Previously, several different conditions have been described according to their appearance (e.g. leukoplakia, kraurosis, lichen sclerosus et vel atrophicus). Owing to the lack of standard criteria much confusion has arisen, and has been compounded by the findings that firstly, all tend to produce an itch-scratch cycle which results in keratinisation, acanthosis, and inflammatory cell infiltration. Secondly, the histological picture may vary from one area of a section to another and features of more than one condition may be present. The current approach is to abandon the previous terms and subdivisions and to classify the changes according to their nature, e.g. degenerative, inflammatory, or dystrophic. A biopsy should include a portion of macroscopically normal tissue.

Dystrophic change may be a precursor of invasive carcinoma. The histological features include irregular morphology, abnormal mitotic activity, and haphazard arrangement of cells. Definite pre-malignant conditions (variously termed 'carcinoma in situ', 'pre-invasive carcinoma', and 'intra-epithelial neoplasia') have been given 'descriptive' eponyms such as Bowen's disease and erythroplasia of Queryrat, but these have no particular merit today.

Paget's disease has the same characteristic histological picture as seen elsewhere in the body. It is a carcinoma of the skin limited to the epidermis. It produces a histological appearance of thickening and infiltration of the epithelium by cells with irregular nuclei and vacuolated cytoplasm.

Vulvectomy is the treatment of choice where pre-malignant conditions are present.

Once the diagnosis of benign vulvitis has been made, therapy can be started. General measures should include advice about local hygiene, adequate rinsing of underwear, and avoidance of local application (deodorants, antiseptics, etc.). Multi-vitamin tablets may help in rare cases of deficiency states. The local measures may be employed if general measures are unsuccessful.

Initially, bland ointments should be used (e.g. zinc and castor oil); mild steroid ointment (0.5% and 1% hydrocortisone) should then be tried and, if these do not alleviate the symptoms, oestrogen creams may be the treatment of choice—especially when there are atrophic changes. As a last resort, surgical measures (such as local denervation of the skin or simple vulvectomy) may be required. However, as the condition may well recur, you must perform full investigations (see above) before embarking on surgery, and this should include taking an expert dermatological opinion.

Comment

Gynaecological symptoms are not always due to local pathology and may reflect systemic disease. This is well exemplified by pruritus vulvae.

Vulval surgery for non-malignant conditions should be performed only as a last resort for symptomatic relief. However, biopsies should be taken in any patient over 50 years of age who has suspicious trophic changes in the vulva. Ulcerated lesions associated with a history of pruritus must be regarded as potentially malignant.

Colposcopy has a definite place in the follow-up and assessment of abnormal vulval epithelium.

Radical vulvectomy is the best treatment for carcinoma of the vulva. Removal of lymph nodes in the inguinal and external iliac groups is essential if recurrence rates are to be reduced. The procedure demands immaculate nursing care and physiotherapy to reduce the risks of sepsis and thromboembolism.

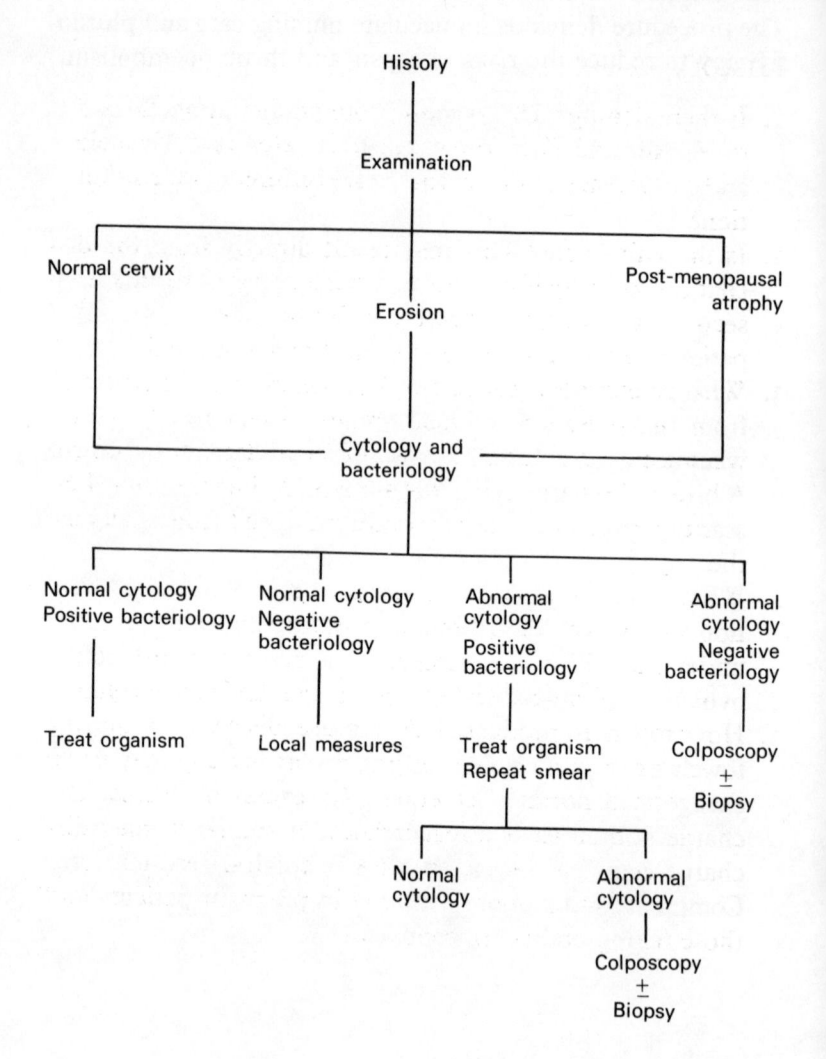

```
                          History
                            |
                       Examination
                            |
        ┌───────────────────┼───────────────────┐
   Normal cervix          Erosion         Post-menopausal
                            |                atrophy
                            |
                      Cytology and
                      bacteriology
                            |
   ┌────────────────┬───────┴────────┬────────────────┐
Normal cytology   Normal cytology   Abnormal         Abnormal
Positive         Negative          cytology         cytology
bacteriology     bacteriology      Positive         Negative
   |                |              bacteriology     bacteriology
   |                |                  |                |
Treat organism   Local measures    Treat organism   Colposcopy
                                   Repeat smear         ±
                                        |            Biopsy
                                  ┌─────┴─────┐
                                Normal     Abnormal
                                cytology   cytology
                                              |
                                          Colposcopy
                                              ±
                                           Biopsy
```

Vaginal Discharge

History

1. Is there itching? This is found commonly in infections due to Monilia and *Trichomonas vaginalis*. However, the colour and consistency of the discharge are different (see Examination).
2. Is the vulva sore? This may result directly from the discharge especially if it is due to Trichomonas or results from secondary infection introduced by scratching. In older patients, a vulval dystrophy should be considered.
3. What colour is the discharge? A brown discharge may result from the presence of blood. Many discharges, however, when exposed to the air may stain the underclothes brown. A brown discharge occurring at monthly intervals may be a scanty period or a scanty withdrawal bleed from hormone therapy.
4. What is the variation? The normal cervical mucus production varies cyclically, becoming watery and more profuse under the action of oestrogen to a maximum just before ovulation, after which it becomes thicker and less in volume.
5. How much is produced? A profuse discharge requiring towels or several changes of underwear per day may be an exaggerated normal 'secretion'. An excess of normal discharge is thus termed leucorrhoea. A similar vaginal discharge may be associated with a cervical 'erosion' (see Comment) and is more common in pregnant patients and those taking oral contraceptives.

Examination

The examination may often reveal diagnostic signs, for example; Monilial infections produce a thick, off-white, cheesy discharge. Trichomonal infections produce marked reddening of the vagina, often with tiny red speckles, and a thin, profuse, frothy yellow-green discharge. Atrophic changes may be seen in the post-menopausal vagina where the normal flora is absent and opportunistic organisms have become established. Cervical 'erosions' may be seen to be the source of a mucoid discharge, which is usually clear or white. In children, check for threadworms.

Management

Specimens are sent for bacteriology and cytology. A high vaginal swab is cultured aerobically and anaerobically. A pipette specimen is taken to look for Trichomonas in a fresh specimen. If a gonococcal infection is suspected, swabs should be taken from the cervical canal, vagina, and urethra, transported in Stewart's medium and cultured anaerobically.

Common organisms are treated as follows:

Monilia. Nystatin pessaries 1 b.d. for 14 days or clotrimazole pessaries two at night for three nights (these are also effective against *Trichomonas vaginalis*). For other agents refer to MIMS or B.N.F.

Trichomonas. Metronidazole 200 mg t.d.s. for 10 days, or 2 g in divided dose over two days. The patient's husband or consort should receive similar simultaneous treatment. Clotrimazole pessaries (as for Monilia). For other agents refer to MIMS or B.N.F.

Staphylococci, Streptococci, coliforms, anaerobes. Triple sulphonamide cream applied b.d. for ten days; metronidazole is effective against anaerobes; clindamycin is effective against bacteriodes.

There is, however, some dispute as to whether finding these organisms is causally related to the discharge and whether treatment is necessary.

If an 'erosion' is present, this may be treated by cryocauterisation or diathermy. The columnar epithelium is destroyed and sloughs over the following 10–14 days and this is associated with an increase in discharge. Thereafter healing occurs with regeneration of squamous epithelium.

In the post-menopausal patient, other signs or symptoms may indicate a need for systemic hormone replacement therapy (HRT), in which case the lowest effective dose should be used. A cyclical regime is often advocated and/or progestogen is given so that, if the endometrial bleeding occurs, it will do cyclically and not lead to diagnostic confusion (see Post-Menopausal Bleeding).

If it is desired to treat the vagina only, an oestrogen-containing cream is used. These produce glycogenation of the vaginal epithelium, allowing lactobacilli to flourish and displace opportunistic organisms. There is a varying degree of systemic absorption from the vagina which may cause endometrial stimulation and bleeding (see Post-Menopausal Bleeding).

Comment

In the reproductive era the natural defences against vaginitis are due to the effects of oestrogen on the vaginal epithelium. Glycogen is present in vaginal squamous epithelium when there is adequate circulating oestrogen and this allows *Lactobacillus acidophilus* to flourish. The normal flora produces a local pH of 4.5 which is hostile to most organisms. Pre-pubertally and post-menopausally this defence is absent and opportunistic infections occur. In these circumstances especially, any foreign body (common in young girls) will cause vaginitis.

Altered local environment due to pregnancy, combined oral contraceptives, or diabetes mellitus leads to an increased incidence of Monilia.

Repeated infections may be due to re-infection from any asymptomatic infection in the male partner. Recurrence merits treatment of the male (particularly in the case of Trichomonas). Repeated recurrences of monilial infection merits a glucose tolerance test. The shorter the course of treatment, the more likely is the patient to comply with advice and complete the course — thus the benefits of the shorter courses described above.

The inexperienced clinician should be wary of vaginal discharge in the elderly or menopausal patient. This should be regarded with suspicion as it may be due to an underlying cervical or endometrial neoplasm or, rarely, carcinoma of the fallopian tube, particularly if the discharge is blood stained.

The symptoms of genital prolapse are often aggravated by a discharge. Appropriate treatment of the discharge may well lead to a marked lessening of the symptoms.

Erosions

The word 'erosion' is included here because of its still widespread use. The term is misleading. The reddened area visible is the transformation zone from squamous to glandular epithelium. This zone is often more prominent in patients who are pregnant or taking combined oral contraceptives. In parous patients, lateral cervical lacerations may allow the cervical lips to pout open revealing more glandular epithelium than usual, this is an ectropion.

Cytology of the Female Genital Tract

The study of exfoliated or desquamated cells from the female genital tract has several clinical applications and the different types of preparations need to be considered. The smears should be made immediately onto the glass slides and fixed, without drying, with 95% ethyl alcohol. After fixation they are stained (usually by a Papanicolaous method) and read.

Cervical smears are usually obtained with an Ayres spatula, although a cotton wool swab moistened with saline is useful if the cervix is 'dry' or atrophic. The smears are used as a screening procedure for pre-malignant conditions of the cervix and may confirm clinical suspicion of frank malignancy.

It should be noted that cytological assessment of smears only reveals *abnormality* of the cells, a definite diagnosis of the degree of abnormality and invasion, if present, requires *histological* examination of either a colposcopic-directed biopsy or a direct-vision 'punch' or 'cone' biopsy.

Endocervical smears can be obtained with an aspiration pipette, and are of value in detecting lesions. They are not widely used.

Vaginal smears obtained from the posterior fornix with a pipette may help in detecting endometrial lesions.

Endometrial smears can be obtained using a special brush and aid the detection of endometrial lesions. The results of these and posterior fornix smears are variable and relatively poor in terms of successful 'pick-up' of abnormalities, thus their application is limited. Vacuum aspiration or diagnostic curettage are preferred.

Lateral wall vaginal smears are obtained from the upper-third of the lateral vaginal wall using a saline-moistened cotton wool swab. Squamous cells of the three layers (superficial, intermediate, and basal) are obtained and their relative numbers are used to assess the patient's hormone status or to monitor hormone treatment. This comparison of the number of each cell type is known as the maturation or karyopyknotic index (KPI).

Abnormal Cervical Cytology

If a cervical 'smear' reveals any abnormality, a further smear should be taken to eliminate the slight possibility of identification error. In the absence of a recognisable clinical lesion it is wise to defer the repeat smear for 4–6 weeks because a small lesion can be removed by the first scrape and false-negative smears can result from taking the second smear before abnormal epithelium has had time to regrow. In the same way, if a woman has had abnormal cytology during pregnancy and her post-natal smear is negative, this should be repeated in three months to check whether or not abnormal epithelium has regrown.

Terminology

The form of the cytology report varies in different hospital laboratories. It can consist of a description of the cells which are present (reactive, dyskaryotic, or malignant), or it may be an interpretation of the whole smear giving the anticipated histological lesion and a recommendation for appropriate action.

At present there are two terminologies in use to describe the histology of pre-invasive lesions of the cervix. The older system uses the terms 'mild dysplasia', 'moderate dysplasia', 'severe dysplasia', and 'carcinoma *in situ*'. This system has the disadvantage that there is an apparent separation between severe dysplasia and carcinoma *in situ*, whereas there are differences of opinion between histopathologists as to which histological pattern would be put into each category. The newer system looks upon the lesion as a continuous spectrum which justifies the term 'Cervical Intra-epithelial Neoplasia' (CIN) and indicates the degree of abnormality by three grades, i.e. CIN I, CIN

Abnormal Cervical Cytology

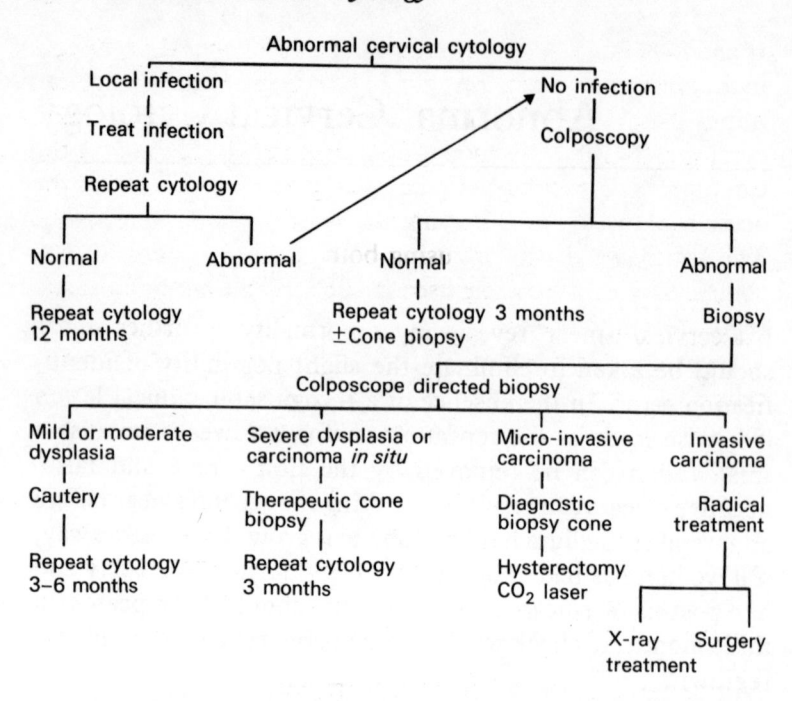

```
                    Abnormal cervical cytology
         ┌──────────────────┴──────────────────┐
   Local infection                         No infection
         │                                     │
   Treat infection                         Colposcopy
         │                                     │
   Repeat cytology                  ┌──────────┴──────────┐
   ┌─────┴─────┐                 Normal                Abnormal
 Normal    Abnormal                 │                     │
   │           │           Repeat cytology 3 months     Biopsy
Repeat     ─────→          ± Cone biopsy
cytology
12 months
              Colposcope directed biopsy
┌──────────────┬───────────────────┬──────────────────┬──────────────┐
Mild or moderate  Severe dysplasia or   Micro-invasive      Invasive
dysplasia         carcinoma in situ     carcinoma          carcinoma
    │                   │                   │                  │
Cautery           Therapeutic cone    Diagnostic           Radical
                  biopsy              biopsy cone          treatment
    │                   │                   │                  │
Repeat cytology   Repeat cytology     Hysterectomy      ┌──────┴──────┐
3–6 months        3 months            CO₂ laser       X-ray       Surgery
                                                      treatment
```

Table 2. Comparison of terminologies used to report abnormal cervical cytology.

	Anticipated/Histology	
DHSS code	Dysplasia/CIS/ Invasive cancer	CIN/Invasive cancer
1. Inadequate specimen	Not relevant	Not relevant
2. Negative	Not relevant	Not relevant
3. Mild dysplasia	Mild dysplasia	CIN I
No code	Moderate dysplasia	CIN II
4. Severe dysplasia/	Severe dysplasia	CIN III
carcinoma *in situ*	Carcinoma *in situ*	CIN III
5. Carcinoma *in situ*/?	Carcinoma *in situ*	CIN III
Invasive	? Micro-invasion	CIN III
	Micro-invasion	Micro-invasion
	Squamous carcinoma (More than 5 mm invasion of stroma)	Squamous carcinoma
6. ? Glandular carcinoma	Adenocarcinoma	Adenocarcinoma

II and CIN III. The disadvantage of this system is that changes in the epithelium due to reaction to infection or local trauma can mimic the changes seen in CIN I and II both histologically and cytologically and the abnormality is not necessarily part of the carcinogenetic pathway. These cases probably account for the occasional cases in which abnormal smears regress to negative. The anticipated histology using both of these systems can be compared with the coding used in the DHSS Cytology request report form as in Table 2.

Confusion can also arise when the cytology report names the cells seen as 'dyskaryotic' or 'malignant'. It is now recommended that the term 'malignant cell' is reserved for smears in which the cytologist is convinced that an invasive cancer is present, although in some laboratories, cells are still referred to as 'malignant' when a severe intra-epithelial lesion is anticipated. In case of doubt it is wise to consult the cytopathologist to establish the implications of the form of report used. It is always useful to do this on moving from one hospital to another.

Management of abnormal smears

Local infection, such as *Trichomonas vaginalis* or Monilia may interfere with the cytological appearances of the smear. You may be able to identify the causative organism on the smear itself but, if not, perform bacteriological examination and give appropriate treatment (see Vaginal Discharge).

Colposcopic examination is an extremely useful aid which enables the colposcopist to examine the cervix in vivo under low-power magnification. The characteristic appearances and vascular patterns aid diagnosis and define abnormal areas from which a biopsy can be taken. The procedure has significantly reduced the number of cone biopsies performed in units where it is used.

Not all units have ready access to a colposcopy service. It is then necessary to determine the degree of the abnormality, and to rule out an invasive lesion by histological examination. Application of an iodine solution (Schiller's test) reveals the abnormal epithelium (normal glycogen-containing squamous cells take up the iodine and stain brown, other cells do not stain) and helps determine biopsy sites. In most units, where colposcopy is not available, cone biopsy is an alternative.

Only *histological examination* can confirm the diagnosis of, and differentiate between in-situ, micro-invasive, and invasive lesions. Usually a cone biopsy is performed. However, a more conservative approach using a colposcopically directed biopsy may be desirable, particularly in young women and cases occurring during pregnancy.

Even if a colposcopy service is available, a cone biopsy is indicated in the following circumstances: 1. When, in the presence of abnormal smears, there is no abnormality seen with the colposcope (the lesions being possibly endocervical); 2. When the whole extent of the lesion cannot be surveyed with the colposcope; 3. When a colposcopically directed biopsy reveals micro-invasion.

Management of abnormal histology

Complete excision of the area in the cone biopsy showing in-situ changes will allow conservative management. This will entail the patient attending for regular cervical smears, supported when necessary by colposcopy, for an indefinite period.

Incomplete excision of the abnormal epithelium may require further excision of the affected area if this is indicated by follow-up cytology. In patients who do not want any more children, a total hysterectomy may be performed, while those who want more children should be treated conservatively using cryocautery, diathermy, or perhaps laser therapy and close follow-up.

Micro-invasive carcinoma (stage 1A) is a lesion confined to the cervix with a stromal invasion. Unfortunately, there is a difference of opinion both as to when a micro-invasive lesion becomes an occult or early invasive lesion and, also as to management. Most authorities in the UK adopt 5 mm as a limit of invasion below which total hysterectomy is considered to be appropriate and beyond which treatment is instigated as for invasive lesions. There is, however, a growing body of opinion which advocates a more conservative approach and the newly-introduced CO_2 laser equipment may have a role here.

Comment

The use of cervical smears to 'prevent' frank carcinoma of the cervix is now well established practice. The use of cone biopsies to confirm the histological diagnosis is not without risk; there are short-term problems of secondary haemorrhage and sepsis, and long-term dangers in subsequent pregnancy of cervical incompetence or stenosis, or of subfertility due to lack of cervical mucus. With its ability to 'recognise' abnormal epithelium and allow direct biopsy, thus limiting excision of tissue, the colposcope should aid in minimising these problems in the future.

Patients with *abnormal* cervical cytology requesting sterilisation may be better treated by total hysterectomy. It is advisable, therefore, to ensure that these patients have a cervical smear taken or that they have had a normal smear report within the previous 18 months.

Summary of management of CIN lesions

CIN I and II. Most lesions are easily surveyed colposcopically: small lesions may be removed with biopsy forceps, larger areas may be destroyed with cryotherapy, diathermy, or CO_2 laser. In a small number of cases conisation may be appropriate. Repeat cytological or colposcopic assessment is carried out after 3-6 months.

CIN III. Management depends upon the extent of the lesion. Once invasion has been excluded, the lesion may be destroyed as for CIN I and II, however, cone biopsy is usually performed. If the patient wishes to be sterilised or is having menstrual problems, total hysterectomy may be preferable. Hysterectomy or laser therapy are indicated if abnormal epithelium remains after treatment. In all cases of in-situ lesions, prolonged follow-up is indicated.

The combination of cytology, colposcopy, and histology in the management of abnormal cervical epithelium has brought a much more scientific approach to the problem and has eliminated many unnecessary cone biopsies with their possible complications.

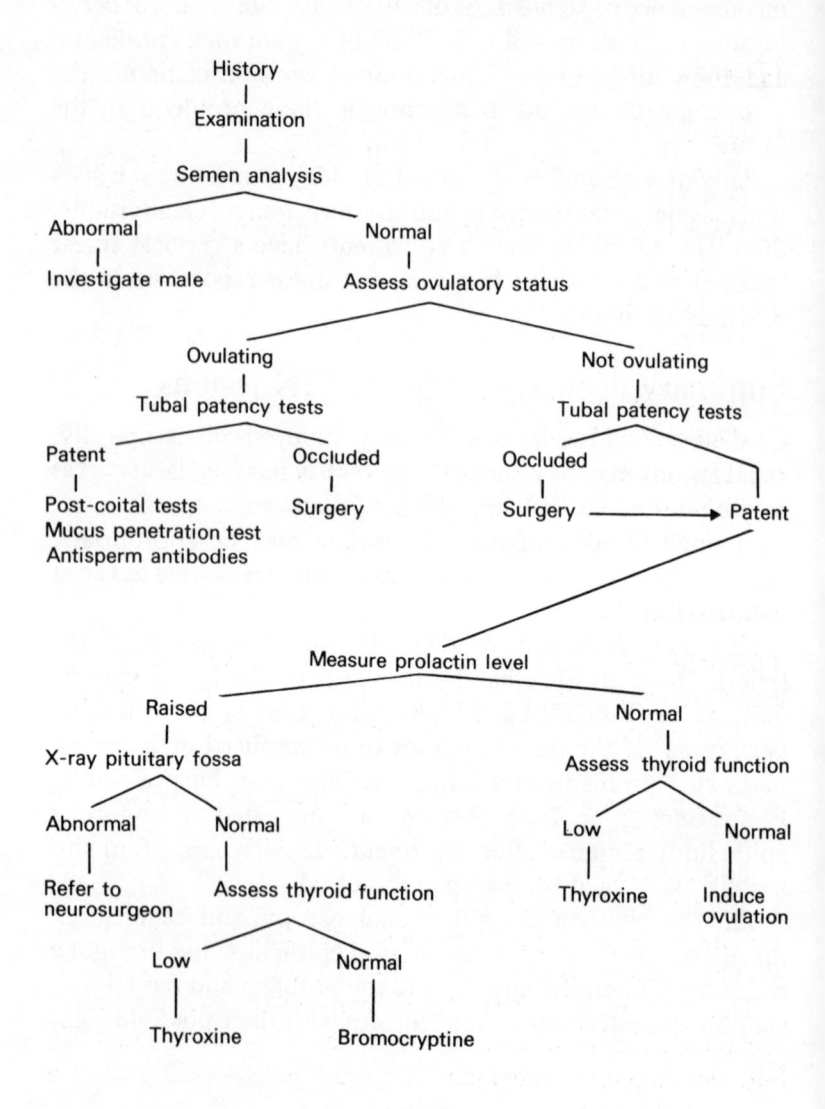

```
                        History
                           |
                      Examination
                           |
                     Semen analysis
                     /           \
              Abnormal           Normal
                 |                  |
         Investigate male    Assess ovulatory status
                              /              \
                        Ovulating          Not ovulating
                            |                   |
                    Tubal patency tests    Tubal patency tests
                      /         \             /          \
                  Patent      Occluded   Occluded       Patent
                    |            |          |
            Post-coital tests  Surgery   Surgery ——→
            Mucus penetration test
            Antisperm antibodies


                          Measure prolactin level
                          /                    \
                      Raised                  Normal
                         |                       |
                 X-ray pituitary fossa   Assess thyroid function
                      /      \                 /         \
                Abnormal    Normal          Low        Normal
                    |          |             |            |
                Refer to   Assess thyroid  Thyroxine    Induce
              neurosurgeon   function                  ovulation
                             /     \
                          Low     Normal
                           |         |
                       Thyroxine  Bromocryptine
```

Subfertility — Female

History
1. Is it primary or secondary infertility? Tubal problems are more likely in secondary infertility, particularly if there has been any puerperal sepsis or problems with pelvic infection.
2. Does the patient have a regular, trouble-free menstrual pattern?
3. Is there any galactorrhoea?
4. Is there a history of pelvic inflammatory disease or appendicitis (both may lead to tubal damage)?
5. Is there any suggestion of thyroid or adrenal dysfunction or diabetes mellitus?
6. How often is intercourse occurring and are there any difficulties?

Examination
The patient should undergo a full, general examination and urinalysis. Particular attention should be paid to the following:
1. The secondary sexual characteristics and their degree of development.
2. The presence of hirsutism which may reflect polycystic ovary syndrome, androgen secreting tumour of the ovary, or adrenal disturbance.
3. Evidence of thyroid dysfunction.
4. The presence of pelvic masses or tenderness.
5. The position, size and mobility of the uterus.

The *semen analysis* should be performed within an hour of the specimen being produced, preferably by masturbation directly into the container provided. It should *not* be collected in a condom. Three days' abstinence from ejaculation should be requested prior to the sample being produced. An abnormal result requires a further specimen for analysis and investigation of the patient's partner (see Subfertility — Male).

Ovulation may be inferred by observing a sustained rise in the basal temperature chart, this follows the increase in metabolic rate which is caused by the progesterone produced by the corpus luteum. You can confirm that ovulation has occurred by histological examination of the pre-menstrual endometrium; this also permits exclusion of tuberculosis of the endometrium. If available, estimation of the serum progesterone level in the luteal phase of the cycle is valuable as is urinary pregnanediol excretion. The presence of a fresh corpus luteum seen at laparoscopy is also confirmatory. Changes in cervical mucus following ovulation include a decrease in volume, decrease in Spinnbarkeit (stretchability), increase in viscosity and absence of 'ferning' on drying.

Tubal patency may be assessed by 1. Chromotubation — dye (methylene blue or indigo carmine) injected through the cervix and passing along the tubes, can be seen at laparoscopy and gives the most useful information about tubal patency; it also allows better assessment of the chances of success of tubal surgery. In the presence of a hydrosalpinx, a co-existing cornual block may be missed and some gynaecologists advise subsequent salpingography to confirm the position before attempting surgery. 2. Salpingography — tubal spasm may give a false result, but this is uncommon under anaesthesia. 3. Gas insufflation — this is associated with a relatively high incidence of misleading results.

A *post-coital test*, if performed correctly around the time of ovulation within four hours of intercourse, will show if the spermatozoa can survive in the cervical mucus. It also confirms adequate coital technique! If the test is repeatedly poor, it may be a result of antisperm antibody activity present in the mucus. In-vitro mucus penetration studies can be performed.

Prolactin levels should be measured and *thyroid function tests* performed as discussed under Amenorrhoea where the exclusion of *drug therapy* is also outlined.

Comment

You should remember that subfertility is a problem of the *couple*. Where possible, both partners should be investigated and dealt with together. Careful discussion and explanation of the tests and their results should help in allaying anxiety. A sympathetic, tactful approach is also essential so that neither partner feels 'to blame' or is left with guilt feelings which in turn lead to marital strife.

Psychological factors play an important part in some cases. This is well exemplified by the number of pregnancies which occur *after* a couple have adopted a child.

Although, for clarity and ease of comprehension, the flow-chart describes the investigations in sequence, in practice many steps are performed concurrently.

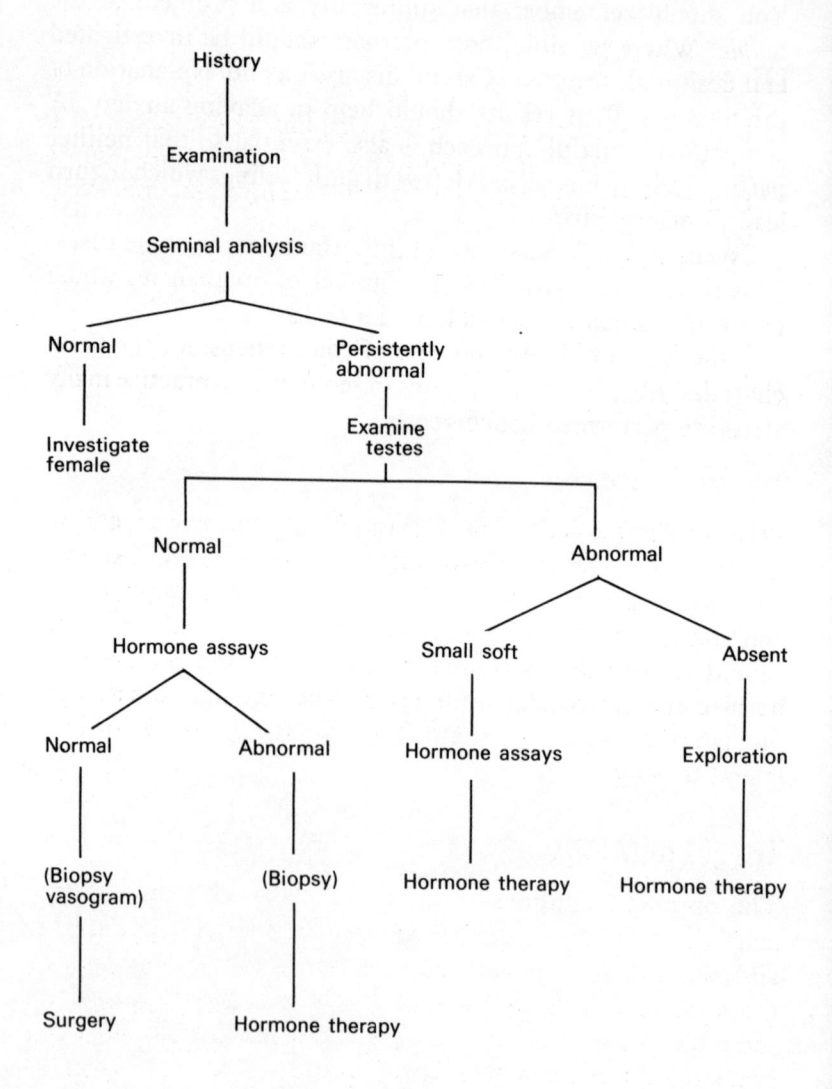

```
History
  |
Examination
  |
Seminal analysis
  /            \
Normal          Persistently
  |             abnormal
Investigate       |
female          Examine
                testes
              /         \
          Normal         Abnormal
            |           /        \
       Hormone assays  Small soft  Absent
         /     \         |          |
     Normal  Abnormal  Hormone    Exploration
       |       |       assays        |
    (Biopsy (Biopsy)     |        Hormone
    vasogram)            |        therapy
       |                 |
       |              Hormone
       |              therapy
    Surgery    Hormone therapy
```

Subfertility — Male

History
1. Is there a *surgical history* such as hernia repair (especially in infancy), torsion of the testes, or late descent of the testes?
2. Is there a medical history of mumps orchitis, tuberculosis, testicular trauma, endocrine or general illness?
3. Has the patient fathered any previous children?
4. Is there a history of impotence, premature ejaculation, or coital difficulties?
5. How often is intercourse occurring? (Two or three times a week is regarded as 'normal'.)

Examination
Perform a full examination, looking for evidence of endocrine disturbance or chronic illness and take particular note of secondary sexual characteristics such as body hair distribution, penis and urethral meatus. The site, size and consistency of the testes should be assessed. Examine the patient for the presence of herniae and varicoceles while he is standing, and palpate the prostate gland by rectal examination with the patient in the left lateral position.

Investigations
The optimal conditions for semen analysis are obtained by collecting a fresh masturbation specimen (after three days' abstinence) in a clean container (*not* a condom). It should be in the laboratory within approximately one hour of production. In some centres split ejaculates are examined for more detailed evaluation. The characteristics of a normal specimen are:

Liquefaction: complete without undue viscosity within 30 minutes.
Volume: 2–5 ml.
Sperm density: more than 40×10^6 motile spermatozoa per ml.
Motility: more than 40% showing progressive forward motility (ranking scales of motility may be used).
Morphology: more than 40% showing normal morphology.
Agglutination: should not be present at one hour after ejaculation.
Fructose: should be present, its absence is associated with congenital bilateral absence of the vasa.

If the specimen is found to be abnormal it should be repeated at least once more after no less than one month. Sperm production is prolific and subject to suppression by even minor transient ailments. As maturation takes approximately three months, there is no point in repeating the analysis too quickly. If repeated analyses are abnormal, proceed according to the clinical findings of testes and hormone analysis.

The results of *hormone assays* may give a prognostic indication of testicular potential:

1. Raised FSH and LH levels reflect testicular failure and are usually associated with small, soft testes.
2. Raised FSH and normal LH levels suggest tubular failure with normal Leydig cell function, the testes are often small and soft but may be clinically normal.
3. Low FSH and LH levels suggest hypothalmic-pituitary malfunction, the testes are usually clinically normal or rarely small. In these patients it is worthwhile performing both a releasing hormone (GnRH) stimulation test and a clomiphene stimulation test to determine if there is a role for long-term therapy.

The significance of hyperprolactinaemia in the male is uncertain; it may be associated with impotence or a high ejaculatory volume.

If the testes are normal in size and the hormone assays are normal, testicular biopsy is indicated. If azoospermia is present, a vasogram may identify the site of blockage. Specialist urological advice is required as reconstructive surgery may be possible.

Testicular biopsy. The role of testicular biopsy in the investigation of male subfertility is disputed. Where the FSH and LH levels are raised, especially if the testes are small and soft, there is no appropriate treatment available. In the presence of normal hormone assays and normal testicular size and consistency, there is usually normal spermatogenesis. Anti-testicular antibodies have been described following testicular biopsy. However, biopsy allows a histological assessment to be made of testicular structure and thus is an index of potential fertility. The appearances often reflect structural changes anticipated from the hormone assays:

1. Primary testicular failure shows a low Johnsen score and, if due to Klinefelter's syndrome, may show the characteristic features of tubular sclerosis and nodular hyperplasia of the Leydig cells. No treatment is applicable.
2. Tubular failure may show either a Sertoli cell-only pattern or a germ cell arrest with normal Leydig cells. No treatment is applicable.
3. With hypothalamo-pituitary malfunction, the histological appearances are of normal testicular structure with a high Johnsen score suggesting a good prognosis.

The Johnsen score is a ranking method of 'quantifying' the histological appearances. The higher the score, the more normal the appearance and the better the prognosis.

Exploration is indicated for the maldescended or ectopic testis which has a much increased risk of undergoing malignant change.

Chromosome karyotyping is not performed routinely owing to a lack of facilities and costs. Unless special banding studies are performed, very few abnormalities are found that cannot be anticipated clinically (e.g. Klinefelter's syndrome).

Therapy

Hormone therapy is indicated in only a few cases. *Gonadotrophins* — only where endogenous levels are low and biopsy shows normal patterns with germ cells. There is *no* indication for empirical gonadotrophin therapy in patients with oligospermia. *Testosterone* — where testes are removed or non-functional, testosterone can be given to maintain normal androgen levels. *Clomiphene* — where the abnormality is a low FSH and LH with a positive clomiphene stimulation test. *Tamoxifen* — an anti-oestrogen which may be used in similar situations to clomiphene. Note that it is common practice to prescribe these agents empirically in cases of oligospermia. Such practice is of no proven value and these drugs should only be used where there is an unequivocal indication.

If the male factor is not remediable the couple may be suitable for donor insemination; this should be arranged only after very careful counselling. Adoption is another alternative, although it is becoming more difficult to adopt these days with better contraceptive facilities and therapeutic abortion being more widely available. Insemination with the husband's own semen (AIH) is applicable for patients with organic impotence, retrograde ejaculation and penile anomalies. In a small number of patients with oligospermia it may be possible to concentrate and store ejaculates for subsequent insemination; however, the results in this group are poor.

Comment

The treatment of male subfertility is inadequate at present. Eventually the couple may be left with the choice of artificial insemination by donor or adoption. Both choices are not without emotional difficulties and the couple should be advised to consider them very carefully before making a decision.

See also Subfertility — Female.

Urinary Symptoms

History

It is notoriously difficult to make an accurate diagnosis in cases of urinary incontinence from the history alone as patients are often unable to give a clear description of the symptoms. However, it is most important that you make an accurate assessment before starting treatment: if the wrong management is undertaken, the situation may be worsened and these ladies are often in a miserable state to begin with.

You should determine whether the incontinence is present all the time (true incontinence), whether it occurs with stimuli such as coughing or straining, or whether it is associated with an intense desire to micturate (urge incontinence). The presence of other associated factors in the history should be sought. *True incontinence* occurs when the patient is always wet (although this may be less noticeable at night when urine may pool in the vagina if the patient sleeps supine); this suggests the possibility of a urinary fistula — the most common in this country being vesico-vaginal. A history of pelvic or vaginal surgery (particularly hysterectomy) or radiotherapy for genital malignancy would be very significant. A vesicovaginal fistula may also follow obstetric trauma (such as improper use of rotational forceps in obstructed labour) which, although rarely seen in this country, is still common in many parts of the world. *Stress incontinence* occurs when the patient strains and the increased intra-abdominal pressure causes a rise in intra-vesical pressure which overcomes the sphincter mechanism. If she strains hard enough, any woman can leak urine but when leakage occurs on minor effort the patient becomes very distressed. A history of difficult labour and multiparity is common and any factor

Urinary Symptoms

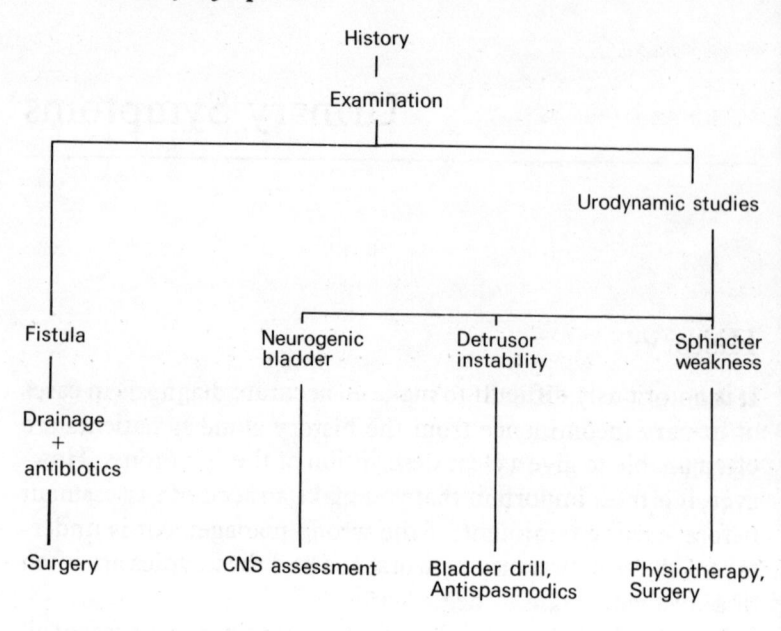

```
                        History
                           |
                      Examination
    _____|_____
    |                |                |                   |
 Fistula       Neurogenic         Detrusor          Urodynamic studies
    |           bladder          instability               |
 Drainage          |                |              Sphincter weakness
    +              |                |                      |
 antibiotics       |                |                      |
    |              |                |                      |
 Surgery      CNS assessment   Bladder drill,       Physiotherapy,
                               Antispasmodics        Surgery
```

which increases intra-abdominal pressure e.g. chronic cough, may contribute. Obese patients have an increased tendency to stress. Leakage may occur with even small volumes of urine in the bladder and there may be no desire to micturate. Urgency of micturition and *Urge incontinence* are associated with an intense and uncontrollable desire to micturate. Associated complaints of frequency and dysuria are not uncommon and suggest 'bladder irritation' (possibly due to infection or oestrogen deprivation). It is important to exclude urinary tract infection in these patients.

The history should also elicit whether there are any neurological symptoms such as visual disturbances, abnormalities of speech or gait and any weakness. Urinary symptoms may be a manifestation of a neurological disease such as multiple sclerosis, where the bladder becomes over-distended and dribbling incontinence occurs. This is due to an 'insensitivity' of bladder nerve endings and/or a failure of normal detrusor muscle activity. The presence of haematuria may reflect a severe infection or a neoplasm.

Examination

A full examination is important. You should note any obesity, evidence of chronic respiratory disease or intra-abdominal mass which may aggravate or provoke stress incontinence. Urinalysis should not be forgotten to exclude infection and also to determine the presence of glucose or protein. Glycosuria due to diabetes may be associated with polyuria and urinary tract infection.

You must perform a *pelvic examination* to exclude any pelvic mass or uterine enlargement, and to look for atrophic changes in the vagina or uterovaginal prolapse. The presence of demonstrable stress incontinence should be sought, and will be better demonstrated in the presence of a full bladder; it is therefore preferable to examine patients complaining of urinary symptoms both *before* and after emptying their bladder. The Sim's speculum is valuable for visualising the anterior vaginal wall to assess the presence of a cystocele or urethrocele, or perhaps a fistula. A fistula may be demonstrated by instilling a solution of methylene blue into the bladder and observing the presence of the dye on swabs suitably placed at different levels in the vagina (three swab test).

When appropriate you should perform a full *neurological examination* including assessment of the sensation of the perineal region, muscle tone, power and reflexes. Include observation of the gait, cerebellar function and optic fundi. This may necessitate admission or referral to a neurologist.

Some objective assessment of the situation may be obtained from a 'bladder chart' where the patient keeps an accurate record of the times at which she micturates and the volume she passes. This is also a useful way of assessing treatment when dealing with detrusor instability. Cystoscopy may be useful in cases where infection or irritation (trigonitis) are suspected and is mandatory in the presence of haematuria. X-ray studies may demonstrate signs suggestive of sphincter weakness (micturating cystogram). IVU studies may be indicated in the presence of a history of recurrent infections. A clean, mid-stream specimen of urine should be sent for bacteriological examination.

Urodynamic studies

In view of the difficulty in obtaining a clear history and the importance of accurate diagnosis before beginning treatment, it is most useful to have some objective measurement of bladder capacity, detrusor activity and urethral function. These investigations include cystometry and urethrometry. Much valuable information may be obtained with relatively simple apparatus; however, some specialised units have cine-video facilities for observing bladder neck activity. In principle, pressure transducers are placed in the bladder and rectum (the latter to record simultaneous changes in intra-abdominal pressure so that a true picture of intra-vesical pressure change can be obtained) and the bladder is slowly filled with water after first measuring any residual urine volume. The resting bladder tone, the volume of water which gives the first desire to micturate (normally 250–300 ml), and then the detrusor activity can be determined as the volume is increased until the patient experiences intense desire to micturate and can hold no more.

By using a urethral device, a pressure profile along the urethral length can be obtained which measures the 'functional length' of the urethra and the maximum 'squeeze' it exerts. In cases of *detrusor instability*, the resting tone may be raised and the desire to void comes with smaller volumes (perhaps only 75 ml). Detrusor activity occurs prematurely and there is an excessive rise in intra-vesical pressure (greater than 15 cm H_2O) as the bladder fills. The capacity may be diminished. In *stress incontinence* the detrusor activity is normal but the 'functional length' of the urethra is shorter than normal and the maximum pressure it exerts is lowered (normally over 45 cm H_2O). In *neurogenic bladders* there is a high residual volume, no real desire to micurate, and erratic ineffectual detrusor activity.

Management

Treatment of a fistula depends on the cause. Post-operative trauma is the most common cause and the first line of management is continuous urethral drainage to keep the bladder empty, and allow it a chance to heal. Antibiotic therapy is often given to minimise the risk of infection. Drainage may be required for several weeks. If spontaneous healing does not occur, then surgical repair is required but should not be undertaken less than three months after the original operation so as to allow post-operative inflammation to resolve. Meticulous attention to detail in surgical technique and post-operative care are required. If a fistula follows radiotherapy or is associated with neoplasia, successful repair is unlikely and some form of urinary diversion (such as an ileal conduit) is often required.

In the presence of a neurogenic bladder with overflow incontinence a full neurological assessment is required with appropriate treatment if a neurological disorder is demonstrated.

In cases of detrusor instability any infection should be eradicated and this may require a long-term antibiotic therapy. Atrophic changes in the vagina suggest oestrogen deprivation which also may affect urinary epithelium; hormone replacement may help in these cases. Anti-spasmodics may bring about marked improvement: flavoxate is widely used in this disorder.

It is often necessary to 're-train' the bladder and some form of bladder drill is helpful, getting the patient to suppress the desire to micturate for increasingly longer periods. Progress is often slow and these patients require a *very* sympathetic and reassuring approach.

The treatment of *stress incontinence* depends on the severity and on the presence or absence of associated factors. If the patient is obese, weight reduction may well be accompanied by a significant improvement in symptoms. Any chronic respiratory problem should be treated as far as possible and any intra-abdominal mass or ascites treated on its own merits. In cases of mild stress, physiotherapy with pelvic floor exercises may well help.

If the primary cause is weakness of the sphincter mechanism associated with anterior vaginal prolapse, surgical management is usually appropriate. Many procedures have been advocated, the most popular are — sub-urethral buttress and anterior colporrhaphy, sling operations (such as Aldridge sling), and suspension operations (such as Marshall-Marchetti). Surgery is only of benefit in the presence of demonstrable sphincter weakness, thus it is important to make sure that this is the patient's problem. The presence of urethral prolapse alone is *not* necessarily an indication for surgery. If detrusor instability is present the treatment is medical (see above). If the patient is unfit for surgery or declines operative repair, anterior wall prolapse with associated stress incontinence may be controlled by a correctly fitted ring pessary.

Comment

Urinary incontinence is a very distressing problem and patients suffering from it require a great deal of support and reassurance. Objective assessment by urodynamic methods greatly improves the success of treatment as it allows a much clearer assessment of the problem and thus correct treatment.

In some patients with resistant or recurrent problems, the advice of a specialist in urinary problems is extremely useful. The misery which these ladies suffer should never be underestimated.

The presence of anterior vaginal prolapse does not in itself indicate the need for surgery; careful assessment of each patient is necessary. Any symptoms of urgency associated with stress incontinence (mixed incontinence) should arouse your suspicion of detrusor muscle instability, and you should avoid surgery until its need is unequivocally and objectively demonstrated.

2. GENERAL TOPICS

HORMONE THERAPY IN GYNAECOLOGY

Menstrual disorders

It is important in patients with menstrual disorders to exclude systemic, endocrine, and uterine disorders before prescribing hormone therapy (see Heavy or Irregular Menstruation and Amenorrhoea). In patients over 45 years or presenting with peri-menopausal menstrual problems you must exclude intrauterine neoplasia by performing curettage. Where general disease or local pathology in the uterus (such as fibroids) are not confirmed, the menstrual abnormality is termed 'dysfunctional'. Dysfunctional uterine bleeding can be divided into ovular and anovular types.

Ovular bleeding

The most common ovular types are epimenorrhoea and epimenorrhagia. In both types the frequency of the period is increased and, in the latter type, there is also increased blood loss at menstruation. The problem would appear to be a disturbance in the ovary resulting in the follicular phase of the cycle being accelerated. Prolonged bleeding or dysfunctional menorrhagia may occur because of irregular shedding of the endometrium before the proper menstrual flow has begun. This is considered to be due to an inadequate hormonal secretion from the corpus luteum which results in premature breakdown and shedding of the endometrium.

Therapy

1. Oestrogen–progestogen preparations.

2. Progestogens, e.g. norethisterone 5 mg t.d.s. on days 5–25 inclusive of the menstrual cycle; dydrogesterone 10 mg b.d. taken similarly.

Anovulatory bleeding

Anovulatory bleeding is a common cause of irregular bleeding in adolescents and in peri-menopausal patients. Prolonged oestrogenic stimulation of the endometrium unmodified by progesterone may produce a cystic glandular hyperplasia of the endometrium. Eventual breakdown of the endometrium causes heavy, *irregular* menstruation — a condition known as 'metropathia haemorrhagica'. In the adolescent these periods are typically painfree and usually occur at long intervals.

Therapy

If the severity of the bleeding merits treatment, this may be directed to two ends.
1. To induce ovulation with a course of anti-oestrogens, (e.g. clomiphene 50 mg daily for five days starting on the fifth day of the cycle).
2. To convert the proliferative endometrium to a secretory pattern by giving oral progestogen in the third or fourth week of a cycle (e.g. norethisterone 5 mg b.d. on days 19–25, or dydrogesterone 10 mg b.d. on days 11–25).

To arrest a heavy anovular loss, a course of progestogen will bring the bleeding under control in 2–3 days; if continued for a total of ten days then stopped, a withdrawal bleed will occur 2–4 days later which should be less heavy and resemble a normal period (e.g. norethisterone 5 mg t.d.s. for ten days).

Dysmenorrhoea (see also p. 37)

Primary or spasmodic dysmenorrhoea, unassociated with organic pelvic disease, only occurs in ovulatory cycles. Ovulation suppression may be achieved by
1. Combined oral contraceptives.

2. Norethisterone 5 mg t.d.s. on days 5–25 of each cycle.
3. Dydrogesterone 10 mg b.d. on days 5–25 of each cycle.

Treatment should be given for 3–6 cycles, then discontinued. If dysmenorrhoea recurs, treatment may be repeated.

Premenstrual syndrome

The premenstrual syndrome is a cause of much distress to many women and produces a variety of symptoms including headaches, bloating, water retention, breast discomfort, and irritability. Its cause is ill-understood but hormone imbalance is generally held to be responsible.

Response to any particular treatment cannot be predicted in an individual patient, thus it is rather empirical. Suggested regimes include:
1. Combined oral contraceptive.
2. Norethisterone 5 mg b.d. or t.d.s. on days 19–25 of each cycle or, if symptoms start earlier, on days 15–25.
3. Dydrogesterone 10 mg b.d. on days 12–25 of each cycle.

Endometriosis

Endometriotic deposits respond to hormonal stimuli as does normal endometrium, and withdrawal bleeding within the deposits causes severe dysmenorrhoea. In pregnancy, the hormonal changes bring about regression of the endometriotic deposits, a similar effect being produced by prolonged high doses of progestogens.

Pseudopregnancy can be induced by oral combined contraceptive, norethisterone 5 mg b.d. or t.d.s. continuously for at least six months, dydrogesterone 10 mg b.d. or t.d.s. on days 5–25 of each cycle. Reduction in FSH and LH secretion can be achieved by danazol 200–800 mg daily in divided doses. Side-effects are common.

The use of hormones demands caution, especially in girls who may think that they are taking an oral contraceptive; an unwanted pregnancy may result.

Hormone Preparations

Norethisterone

This is a synthetic progestogen which is orally active. Intermenstrual bleeding can be abolished by increasing the dosage but larger doses may result in amenorrhoea. The main side-effects are nausea and weight gain, and exacerbation of migraine and epilepsy may be problems in patients who suffer from these conditions.

Dydrogesterone

This is an orally active progestogen which has no oestrogenic, androgenic, or corticoid properties, unlike most other progestogens. It has no adverse effects on blood clotting and liver function. It does *not* normally inhibit ovulation, so cannot be used as a contraceptive. This property makes it particularly useful in the treatment of endometriosis. There are few side-effects although some patients may complain of breakthrough bleeding, depression, and weight gain.

Danazol

This is an anti-gonadotrophic agent which is administered orally. The dosage should be altered according to the response and is usually in the range of 200–800 mg daily in divided doses. Side-effects are common and include acne, fluid retention, and mild hirsutism — all of which are attributable to the drug's androgenic activity. If these masculinising effects occur, the drug should be stopped immediately. The tendency to produce fluid retention poses a problem when prescribing the drug for cardiac and renal cases. Some patients find the drug difficult to tolerate because of nausea. Administration of danazol may therefore have to be given initially in small divided doses and increased gradually. Danazol may potentiate the action of anticoagulants, so extra caution and close monitoring of the clotting factors are necessary.

Endometrial carcinoma

The use of progestogens in the treatment of carcinoma of the endometrium is controversial. Some success has been claimed by workers in the treatment of vault and pulmonary metastases. The well differentiated adenocarcinomata seem to be the most likely histological group to respond to this treatment. However, the actual value of the therapy remains unproven. High-dose progestogen therapy may be used firstly as an adjunct to surgery given pre- and post-operatively to prevent spread at operation (e.g. gestronol hexanoate 200–400 mg i.m. every five days for 12 weeks or medroxy progesterone acetate 100 mg b.d. or t.d.s. daily for three months); secondly, alone or in conjunction with radiotherapy or cytotoxic agents in patients unfit for surgery or with inoperable lesions (dosage as above but for indefinite duration); thirdly for treating existing metastases (dosage as above), duration depends on whether metastases are hormone responsive. A minimum of eight weeks' therapy should be given.

Progestogen therapy is occasionally used in combination with cytotoxic agents in the management of endometrioid carcinoma of the ovary.

Habitual Abortion

Some authorities believe that progesterone deficiency is a cause of early abortion and habitual abortion. Progesterone is necessary for implantation and maintaining the early gestation. However, it is difficult to prove that progesterone deficiency is the cause and not merely the effect of the at risk pregnancy. Depot progesterone therapy has been advocated in cases of habitual abortion.

Typical regimes are: hydroxyprogesterone hexanoate 250–500 mg i.m. per week up to the 20th week, of dydrogesterone 10 mg b.d. orally continuously to the 20th week.

The use of progestogens may produce masculinisation of the female fetus. They may also prolong a dead pregnancy and result in a missed abortion.

The importance of human chorionic gonadotrophin (hCG) in maintaining the corpus luteum is well known. This has led to hCG being given intramuscularly for habitual abortions. Some authorities advocate 5000 IU of hCG twice weekly to the 20th week, but as yet, there is no satisfactory evidence as to its efficacy.

Hormone Replacement Therapy (HRT) for Climacteric Symptoms

The menopause or problems due to climacteric changes are associated with severe symptoms in approximately 25% of women. Oestrogen replacement therapy as a panacea for the problems of middle-aged women (over 45 years) is to be strongly discouraged. In fact, it is the inappropriate use of oestrogen therapy which has provoked such controversy in recent years.

The menopause occurs when women are about 50, which is a stressful time in a woman's life: she may have problems with teenage offspring or elderly parents, there may be bereavements in the family, or her children have married and left home. Added to this is the feeling she is getting old, and the awareness that she is at the end of her reproductive life. Your treatment should reflect an awareness that the patient is an individual with specific problems and not just a 'case' undergoing the menopause. A reassuring, sympathetic conversation is often better therapy than the oestrogen!

The common symptoms associated with the climacteric are hot flushes, night sweats, loss of libido, dry vagina and dyspareunia, urethral symptoms, urgency of micturition, tiredness and anxiety symptoms. A careful history and assessment of the symptoms must be made. She should be examined thoroughly including breasts, blood pressure, abdomen and pelvis. Take a cervical smear and look for evidence of pelvic pathology, such as uterine or ovarian enlargement. Test the patient's urine for glucose and protein. In patients with an irregular or abnormal peri-menopausal menstrual pattern, a curettage should be performed before beginning hormone therapy.

The method of oestrogen administration should avoid prolonged stimulation of the endometrium and hence endometrial hyperplasia, by provoking scheduled withdrawal bleeds, similar to those of the oral contraceptive pill. This can be achieved by combining a progestogen with the oestrogen in the third week of the cycle. For long-term HRT, to prevent osteoporosis and coronary artery disease, the withdrawal bleeding may be timed at regular intervals. A similar regime may be employed in cases who have undergone bilateral oophorectomy. In posthysterectomy cases, the oestrogen may be given unopposed and continuously. There are several oestrogen-progestogen preparations available but we have found the 1 mg oestradiol valerate and 0.25 mg norgestrel combinations to be particularly effective. The few patients who fail to tolerate this combination, often respond to a change in hormone such as piperazine oestrone sulphate and norethisterone. There is therefore a variable patient response, again similar to that found in oral contraceptives. Poor tablet takers may prefer an oestrogen implant, inserted into the anterior abdominal wall, which is replaced at three-monthly intervals or with recurrence of symptoms.

The *contra-indications* to oestrogen therapy are: a past history or thrombo-embolism or cerebrovascular disease; liver disease; sickle cell anaemia and cases with oestrogen-dependent tumours (breast and uterus). Special caution should be exercised when prescribing oestrogens to patients with diabetes mellitus and hypertension. Whilst the patient remains on oestrogen therapy, she should have her blood pressure and urine checked at six-monthly intervals and her breasts and pelvic organs, together with a cervical smear, checked annually. Intermenstrual or bleeding per vaginam, other than at the expected 'withdrawal bleed' times, should be considered a serious symptom warranting an urgent curettage to exclude intra-uterine pathology.

DRUGS IN GYNAECOLOGY

Antibiotics

Infections of the female genital tract are a common gynaecological problem. The main organisms causing puerperal and post-abortal sepsis are *Escherichia coli*, Gram-negative bacilli, Clostridia, Streptococci and Straphylococci. Pelvic sepsis of uncertain aetiology may be due to gonorrhoea or tuberculosis. Recent studies have shown *Chlamydia trachomatis* to be the underlying organism in many cases of non-gonococcal salpingitis. Some workers have also suggested that *Mycoplasma hominis* may be implicated in pelvic inflammatory disease. In clinical practice therefore, culture of the organisms may be difficult. However, where possible, specimens from the site of infection should be sent to the bacteriologist for culture and testing of sensitivity. The prescribing of broad-spectrum antibiotics blindly should be deprecated, except where the patient's clinical condition demands urgent treatment.

Ampicillin, cotrimoxazole, sulphonamides and *tetracycline* are effective against coliform organisms and some Gram-positive cocci. *Pseudomonas pyocyanea* and Proteus organisms are often resistant to these antibiotics. Infections by these resistant organisms would require treatment with cephalosporins or gentamicin. Caution must be exercised in the use of these drugs especially in cases with impaired renal function because gentamicin can be ototoxic and nephrotoxic. To avoid these serious side-effects, the blood levels of the antibiotics are monitored.

Clindamycin is valuable in the treatment of infections due to Gram-positive organisms and bacteroides. The most serious side-effect of this drug is colitis and, if this occurs, the drug should be discontinued.

Erythromycin has recently gained popularity in the treatment of salpingitis because of its effectiveness against a wide range of organisms: Gram-positive cocci, Mycoplasma L forms, *Haemophilus influenzae*, Chlamydia, Clostridia, Neisseria and *Treponema pallidum*. The drug is contraindicated in patients with a history of hepatic dysfunction.

Metronidazole is active against Trichomonal and anaerobic infections. The usual dose is 200 mg t.d.s. orally for 10 days. However, for Trichomonas infections, a short vigorous course can be given — 2 g over two days — which increases patient compliance. The patient's consort should be treated at the same time to avoid re-infection. Careful explanation is necessary to ensure that the patient and her partner do not misunderstand the nature of the condition and think they have a serious venereal disease. However, the possibility of a coexisting gonococcal infection should be considered, especially in high-risk cases such as patients with signs and symptoms suggestive of pelvic sepsis. The drug can be given prophylactically to reduce anaerobic infections in gynaecological surgery and may be administered rectally by suppositories when the patient is not tolerating oral fluids. For severe anaerobic infections and bacteraemias, the drug may be given intravenously 500 mg/100 ml, eight hourly.

The main *side-effects* include furred tongue, nausea, and gastrointestinal upsets. It is recommended that patient avoid alcohol during the treatment.

The long acting penicillins (e.g. procaine penicillin) are still effective and are the treatment of choice for gonorrhoea and syphilis. In severe acute gonococcal salpingitis, intravenous benzyl penicillin is the preferred treatment.

Anti-Fungal Agents

Clotrimazole

This is effective against Monilia and Trichomonas; it is available as a cream for topical application and vaginal tablets. A big advantage of this agent is the short treatment regime — two vaginal tablets per day for only three days — but some authorities prefer to prescribe it for 5–6 days, as patients often discontinue therapy early anyway, when they have achieved symptomatic relief.

Nystatin

This is a fungicide which is effective against Monilia. It is poorly absorbed from the intestine. Local treatment is by pessary — one twice daily for 14 days — and an ointment and cream are available. It tends to stain the underclothes and the prolonged course is often associated with poor patient compliance.

In recurrent monilial infections, an oral suspension of nystatin together with pessaries will eradicate any reservoir of fungi in the bowel and vagina.

Miconazole

This is an agent effective against fungal and Gram-positive bacterial infections. The drug may be administered as a non-staining pessary, an intra-vaginal cream, or a tampon. The tampon may prove valuable for treatment of monilial infections during menstruation. It is at this time that the patient may have some symptomatic relief due to change in vaginal pH. She is therefore liable to discontinue her treatment prematurely and subsequently get a recurrence of the infection. Anti-fungal treatment, in the form of a tampon, should prevent this problem and be acceptable to the patient during menses.

Fertility Drugs

Bromocryptine

This is an alkaloid analogue of prolactin inhibitory factor (PIF) and is used to lower prolactin levels in cases of hyperprolactinaemia following appropriate investigation (see Amenorrhoea). About one-third of patients presenting with hyperprolactinaemia and amenorrhoea will be found to have a pituitary tumour, usually a chromophobe adenoma. It is therefore mandatory to X-ray the pituitary fossa before beginning bromocryptine therapy. Most of these tumours are less than 1 cm in diameter but they may enlarge during pregnancy and cause pressure on the optic chiasma.

The optimum dosage is 7.5–10 mg daily in divided doses, but this dose is achieved gradually starting with 2.5 mg daily and increasing the dose at weekly intervals, since nausea is a common, though transient, side-effect. Other minor side-effects, such as postural hypotension and nasal congestion, also tend to disappear after a few days. More serious adverse effects, such as confusion, hallucinations, and dyskinesis are fortunately uncommon in the dosages usually used.

In approximately 90% of cases, ovulation and hence menstruation will be occurring regularly within twelve months on dosages between 2.5 and 10 mg per day.

Bromocryptine should only be given under strict supervision and alcohol should be avoided as it potentiates the nausea. The therapy is usually discontinued when pregnancy occurs, although there is no evidence that the drug has any teratogenic properties.

Clomiphene

This is a non steroidal agent with anti-oestrogenic properties, which is used to induce ovulation. Its action is to compete with oestrogen receptor sites in the hypothalamus and anterior pituitary gland and, by doing so, to interfere with the negative-feedback effect of endogenous oestrogens on the hypothalamus and anterior pituitary and so result in an increased secretion of FSH and LH. This is shown by rises in gonadotrophins and oestradiol secretion. The drug is therefore only effective when the hypothalamo-pituitary axis is functional and the ovaries are 'responsive' to endogenous gonadotrophins.

Clomiphene is particularly useful in the treatment of polycystic ovary syndrome, secondary oligomenorrhoea or amenorrhoea of uncertain aetiology, and post-pill amenorrhoea.

Clomiphene citrate is usually taken orally in a dose of between 50 and 150 mg per day for five days (such as days 2–6 inclusive of the menstrual cycle if menstruating). The expected time of ovulation is 7–16 days after beginning therapy. The timing of intercourse should coincide with this. Ovulation can also be confirmed by measurement of the serum progesterone 21 days after starting the drug. In cases where there is a follicular response but no ovulation (shown by a rise in oestradiol but not progesterone, menstruation in amenorrhoeic cases, and a monophasic temperature chart), an intramuscular injection of hCG 14 days after the clomiphene may be given to supplement a deficient mid-cycle LH surge.

Misuse of this drug is common; there is little purpose in using high doses if ovulation occurs with low amounts. The patient should be seen regularly in the gynaecological clinic to check for ovarian enlargement and, in amenorrhoeic cases, to exclude pregnancy. You should exercise caution if there is any ovarian enlargement or Stein-Leventhal syndrome, as ovarian cysts and ovarian 'accidents' may be provoked. Hot flushes are a symptom in about 10% of cases but more serious side-effects, such as blurring of vision, nausea, and vomiting, are uncommon. Twin pregnancy occurs in approximately 10% of cases.

The marked discrepancy between the ovulation and pregnancy rates from clomiphene may be partly explained by the anti-oestrogenic effect on the endometrium and cervical mucus.

Tamoxifen

This is an anti-oestrogen which is used for similar indications and in a similar manner to clomiphene. The dose is 20–80 mg daily for five days.

Gonadotrophins

These are used to stimulate ovulation in cases of hypothalmo-pituitary failure and cases which fail to respond to anti-oestrogens or, where appropriate, bromocryptine. Exogenous FSH and LH are available in the form of human menopausal gonadotrophin. Ovulation is induced, after follicular maturation, with hCG given intramuscularly. Dosage regimes are beyond the scope of this book but close monitoring of the oestrogen response is mandatory to prevent hyperstimulation which may result in ovarian enlargement, ascites, shock, or multiple births.

Uterine Muscle Stimulants (Oxytocics)

Oxytocin

This is a synthetic analogue of the posterior pituitary hormone which is used to produce rhythmic uterine contractions. In gynaecology it is used to stimulate contractions in cases of abortion or after termination of pregnancy. It may be given intravenously as a bolus of ten units or by infusion in 5% dextrose.

Oxytocin is a vasodilator and has properties similar to antidiuretic hormone. Excessive use can therefore result in fluid retention and oedema; cases of water intoxication and cerebral oedema have been reported.

Ergometrine

This is an alkaloid ergot agent which stimulates a tonic contraction in the pregnant uterus. It is particularly useful in arresting uterine haemorrhage after abortion. It may be administered orally or, more usually, parenterally. In emergency, an intravenous injection of 0.5 mg takes effect within 60 seconds.

Ergometrine is a vasoconstrictor and is better avoided in cardiac and hypertensive patients. It may provoke nausea, vomiting, and muscle spasms with numbness in the fingers and toes.

Prostaglandins

These are unsaturated fatty acid derivatives of prostanoic acid which were originally discovered in the prostatic secretions, hence their name. There are about 20 prostaglandins, some are efficient abortifacients, especially E2, which may be administered to induce second trimester abortions or delivery of a late missed abortion. They may be given by intra-amniotic, extra-amniotic or intravenous routes, but the latter is associated with a high incidence of unpleasant side-effects, which include nausea, vomiting, diarrhoea, hyperpyrexia, and local tissue reaction.

The local tissue reaction or 'chemical' phlebitis can be minimised by administering the drug intravenously through an infusion catheter and using an antihistamine, such as chlorpheniramine.

Fewer side-effects are experienced by intra or extra-amniotic infusion. Prostin E2 should be given cautiously to patients who have glaucoma or asthma.

CONTRACEPTION

Many patients require contraceptive advice. Despite widespread publicity and ready access to family planning clinics, there is still a marked ignorance of contraceptive techniques and aids. The gynaecologist should discuss the available methods with the patient so that the most appropriate method for each individual case may be agreed on.

Often patients are referred to the clinic with a request for sterilisation. It is necessary to determine if sterilisation is the most appropriate method of contraception for the patient; in many cases the patient is unaware of available — and perhaps preferable alternatives.

There are six techniques commonly used in the UK beside the pill. The relative efficacity of the different methods is shown in Table 3.

Rhythm method or safe period

This method is the only one acceptable to the Roman Catholic Church and requires a good deal of instruction and motivation. It assumes that the ovum is capable of being fertilised for a short time only (less than 24 hours) and that ovulation occurs 14 days before menstruation. In patients with a regular cycle it is therefore thought possible approximately to determine the day of ovulation. To allow for minor variations in the time of ovulation it is usual to advise the couple to refrain from intercourse for five days before and five days after the anticipated day of ovulation. Apart from the artificial situations imposed by this ten day abstinence, additional problems occur in patients with irregular cycles and in those occasional patients in whom ovulation can be precipitated by their emotional state. Additional

Table 3. Relative efficacy of different contraceptive techniques in order of reliability

Method	Pregnancies per 100 women years
Oral contraception	
combined	0.2–0.5
progestogen	0.5–1.5
IUCD	0.5–5.0
Sheath	10–18
Sheath with spermicide	6–10
Cap	12–20
Cap with spermicide	6–12
Withdrawal	16–22
Spermicide alone	22–25
Safe period	23–28

Note. This table is a composite of quoted figures from several sources and is intended to give a broad comparison between methods. Different figures may be quoted in individual publications.

information regarding the occurrence of ovulation may be obtained by the use of a basal temperature chart.

Withdrawal methods

This is one of the most widely used methods and relies upon variants of firstly, withdrawal prior to orgasm with ejaculation outside the vagina, secondly, withdrawal well before orgasm with no ejaculation, or thirdly, intercourse between the thighs with no vaginal penetration. These methods call for motivation, determination, and timing! They are not very reliable.

Condom

The condom or sheath offers some protection against venereal infection, is also devoid of side-effects, is readily available, and disposable. Unfortunately it requires fitting to the erect penis before intercourse and removal immediately after ejaculation whilst the penis is still erect; this interferes with spontaneity. Another drawback is the decrease in sensitivity for both partners.

Occlusive caps

Latex caps are available which either fit over the cervix or across the vaginal vault (diaphragm) and are designed to prevent spermatozoal access to the cervix. They should be filled with a spermicidial foam or cream for added protection. They are fitted before intercourse and left in situ for at least eight hours afterwards to ensure that the spermatozoa which reach the spermicide are killed. As with condoms, they are free from side-effects but may interfere with spontaneity. They do not interfere with sensitivity for either partner.

Chemical spermicides

The more widely used agents are phenyl mercuric acetate and derivatives of ricinoleic acid and hexylresorcinol. They are available as pessaries, jellies, foams and creams. They should not be used alone, but in conjunction with caps and sheaths.

Intra-uterine devices (IUD, IUCD, coil)

The precise mode of action of these plastic devices is uncertain. They prevent implantation of the fertilised ovum by local effect on the endometrium, perhaps related to prostaglandin release. They are available in a variety of shapes and sizes, and the more recent versions have an additional active agent — copper — in the form of a thin wire wrapped around the stem of the device. This offers additional protection by direct action on the endometrium and cervical mucus.

On a population basis IUCDs are quite attractive: they combine reliability with a 'one time' application (or every two years for the 'active' devices) and low incidence of side-effects. The physical presence of a foreign body in the uterus may lead to expulsion in a few cases, colicky dysmenorrhoea, heavier menstrual losses, and occasionally pelvic sepsis. They are not the method of choice for patients with heavy periods or a history of pelvic inflammatory disease. The use of coils in cases with valvular heart disease is controversial. There is a theoretical risk of bacterial endocarditis which has led to some authorities prescribing antibiotic cover. We prefer to avoid using the coil in these cases. Although smaller models are available for nulliparous patients, there is the risk of pelvic sepsis and salpingitis which may be a relative contraindication in these cases.

Coils have a thread which passes through the cervix and enables one to check that the device is still in situ; should the thread not be visible, an X-ray will determine whether the coil has come out, as they are radio-opaque. Occasionally devices will be found outside the uterus within the peritoneal cavity; this is probably due to incorrect insertion with uterine perforation. Retrieval of inert coils can be achieved by laparoscopy. Copper coils often require laparotomy.

It should be emphasised that the insertion of an IUCD is a skilled technique.

Oral Contraceptives

There are a great many preparations currently available and it is advisable for you to become familiar with just a few of these since one of three or four types will usually suit the needs of the large majority of your patients. Two categories of oral contraceptive exist: the combined oestrogen-progestogen pill, and progestogen only.

Oestrogen-progestogen contraceptives

Combined oral contraceptives act by inhibiting ovulation at hypothalamic level, where the oestrogen suppresses release of FSH and, in concert with progesterone, of LH. The endometrium becomes thin and hypoplastic, the cervical mucus becomes thick, tenacious and resistant to spermatozoal penetration. Tubal transport of the ovum is also affected.

The potentially serious side-effects (see p. 105) appear to be related to the oestrogen component and the daily amount of oestrogen should be no more than 50 μg. Of the numerous combinations available, many contain much lower amounts of oestrogen.

There exists a number of absolute and relative contraindications to the oestrogen component:

Absolute

A history of thrombo-embolic disease
Impaired hepatic function
Pituitary dysfunction
Hormone-dependent tumours
Undiagnosed irregular vaginal bleeding
Potential drug interactions (see below)

Table 4. Drug interactions with oral contraceptives.

Interactions that reduce or may reduce contraceptive efficacy	Interactions that may potentiate the effect of the other drug (*either its pharmacological action or its side-effects*)

Analgesics
  aminodopyrine
  ethylmorphine
  oxyphenbutazone
  phenacetin
  phenazone
  phenylbutazone
Anticonvulsants
  *hydantoins
  *ethosuximide
  *primidone
Anti-infective agents
  *ampicillin
  *chloramphenicol
  neomycin
  nitrofurantoin
  penicillin
  *rifampicin
  *sulphamethoxypyridazine
Hypnotics
  *barbiturates (especially methylphenobarbitone)
  chloral
  dichloralphenazone
  ethchlorvynol
  methaqualone
Tranquilizers
  *chlordiazeproxide
  *chlorpromazine
  *meprobamate
	Analgesics
	  pethidine
	  phenylbutazone
	Antihypertensives
	  reserpine
	Corticosteroids
	Haemostatics
	  aminocaproic acid
	Sedatives
	  chloriazepoxide
	  chlorprothixene
	
	Interactions that may decrease the therapeutic effect of the other drug
	Anticoagulants (all)
	Antidepressants
	  tricyclic compounds
	Antihypertensives
	  guanethidine
	  methyldopa
	Hypoglycaemic agents
	  insulin
	  oral hypoglycaemic agents

* Pregnancies have been reported following interactions with these drugs.

Relative

Hypertension
Migraine
Diabetes mellitus
Uterine fibroids
Epilepsy
Benign breast cancer
Gall bladder disease
History of cholestatic jaundice of pregnancy
Lactation
Heavy smoking (over 20 cigarettes per day, especially if over 35 years of age)
Sickle cell anaemia

If patients are taking other drugs, interactions may occur which may result in: reduction of contraceptive efficiency, potentiation of the effects of the other drug, or reduction in the therapeutic effect of the other drug (Table 4).

Minor side-effects

Many minor side-effects have traditionally been attributed to the components of the pill (see Table 5). Nevertheless, the present view is that the side-effects are not so clear cut.

Should a patient complain of any minor effects after, say three cycles (to allow her body to adjust) you should consider changing the preparation (see Table 6).

Table 5. Minor side effects of oral contraception.

Oestrogenic effects	Progestogenic effects
Fluid retention	Acne, greasy hair
Nausea and vomiting	Increased appetite and gain in weight
Headaches	
Premenstrual irritability	Leg cramps
Cervical erosion	Decreased libido
Tiredness	Breast discomfort
Hypertension	Dry vagina
Mucoid discharge	

Table 6. Suggested action in the event of minor side-effects.

Side-effect	Action
Acne Leg cramps Loss of libido Breast discomfort	Select a preparation with a lower progestogen content
Non-specific headache Nausea Premenstrual tension Mucorrhoea 'Bloating'	Select a preparation with a lower oestrogen content
Migraine	Stop the pill immediately

Effects on bleeding

Heavy bleeding is unusual and should respond to a higher proportion of progestogen. Breakthrough bleeding is not uncommon in the first two cycles but, if it persists after three cycles, a preparation with a higher progestogen content should again be prescribed. This bleeding also occurs in some patients on very low doses of oestrogen and, in this case, a preparation with a higher oestrogen content may rectify the situation. If breakthrough bleeding still persists, full gynaecological assessment is mandatory.

Amenorrhoea whilst taking the pill is a cause of anxiety to the patient and may be caused by too much progestogen or too little oestrogen. Appropriate changes may be made after exclusion of pregnancy.

Combined contraceptives and surgery

There appears to be an increased risk of post-operative deep vein thrombosis amongst women using the combined pill, and it is therefore advisable that oral contraception should be stopped at least two weeks before elective surgical procedures. In emergency situations when the contraception is continued until the time of operation, the prophylactic use of subcutaneous calcium heparin may be considered until the patient is fully ambulant.

Major side-effects

Thrombo-embolism. This is age related and also significantly related to smoking more than 15 cigarettes per day. There is between a five and sixfold increased risk of deep vein thrombosis in pill users. Those over the age of 40 years have an excess mortality of 54.6 per 100 000: 3.3 attributable to the pill, 8.5 to smoking and 42.8 to the combined effects.

Hypertension. The incidence of hypertension is increased between two and threefold in pill users; the increase in blood pressure is usually reversible within a few months of discontinuing the pill.

Stroke. The incidence of stroke is increased by up to threefold, particularly in smokers and hypertensive patients.

Cholecystitis and cholelithiasis. There is a twofold increase in the incidence of these conditions among pill users. The incidence of stones rises with duration of therapy up to five years. The cause is thought to be related to oestrogen-induced alterations in the composition of the bile.

Failure

Pregnancies occurring whilst on the oral contraceptive pill are often due to failure to follow the instructions or simply forgetting to take the tablet. Disturbances of the gastro-intestinal tract such as gastro-enteritis or malabsorption states may also be responsible for failed oral contraception.

Monitoring of patients

Patients should be prescribed the combined oral contraceptive only after careful assessment and exclusion of contraindications. Thereafter they should be seen at twice-yearly intervals for measurement of the blood pressure, urine testing, and breast palpation. The appearance of any of the conditions deemed to be absolute or relative contra-indications to continued therapy should be carefully sought.

Current evidence does not suggest that any benefit is to be gained from temporary cessation of oral contraception ('rest periods').

Progestogen-only contraceptives

Progestogen-only oral contraceptives act by the progestogenic effects on the endometrium and cervical mucus (and possibly tubal function) described above. Ovulation is not reliably suppressed. These agents are taken continuously, rather than the cyclical regimen of the combined pill. They have a higher incidence of unwanted pregnancy (comparable with that due to intra-uterine devices) and also a higher incidence of breakthrough bleeding. Efficacy also falls markedly if the tablets are forgotten. They are best used for patients who are lactating (as oestrogen-containing preparations suppress lactation) and in patients for whom oestrogens are contra-indicated. The progestogen-only pill is a useful contraceptive whilst patients are lactating since, unlike the combined pill, it does not reduce milk production and has no apparent effects on the infant.

A depot injectable form of progestogen-only contraceptive is available. It offers protection for some three months and is useful post-partum when the patient requires rubella vaccination. It suffers from a relatively high incidence of irregular breakthrough bleeding. It has not yet been approved for long-term use by the Committee for Safety of Medicines.

*Much of the material in this section originally appeared in *The Practitioner*. It is reproduced here by kind permission of the Editor.

Conclusion

The choice of contraception is, finally, a personal decision for the patient to take and she should never be 'pressured' into using a method about which she has reservations. It is the gynaecologist's role to inform and, where necessary, reassure her about the contraceptives available.

GYNAECOLOGICAL OPERATIONS — PRACTICAL ASPECTS

Whenever an operation is advised, however minor, it should be remembered that, to the patient, it is a highly stressful ordeal. It is essential to discuss and fully explain the following points:
1. What operation you are advising.
2. Why you are advising it.
3. What the operation will achieve and, equally important, what it will not achieve.
4. What side-effects may be expected, both short and long-term. (Remember that the patient may well have unvoiced fears which you should dispel).
5. What the post-operative course and convalescent period will be.
6. When she will be able to return to her former occupation.
7. What the subsequent out-patient follow-up will be.

It is also useful if these points can be covered, *in an easily understood form*, on a printed sheet given to the patient which she can study at leisure and discuss with her husband.

Although most aspects of practical patient management are learned at the bedside, you should also bear in mind the following: all operations require the written, informed consent of the patient; all patients should have their haemoglobin measured, and non-Caucasian patients should have haemoglobin electrophoresis performed. All surgical specimens should be sent for histological examination.

The histological or specimen forms vary from hospital to hospital. It is important, however, in gynaecological specimens to include details of the patient's LMP and, where relevant, menstrual cycle. If a malignancy is suspected, as in PMB, the form should be marked **URGENT**.

Abdominal Procedures

Hysterectomy

In these women, pregnancy must be excluded, particularly in cases with irregular periods. Two units of whole blood should be cross-matched and available. See comment about obtaining the husband's consent under Sterilisation.

If bilateral oophorectomy is also performed, hormone replacement therapy may well be required subsequently.

The usual post-operative stay is 7–10 days and the follow-up out-patient visit is six weeks after the operation.

Myomectomy

Two units of whole blood should be cross-matched for the operation. As myomectomy can be technically difficult and haemorrhagic, it is advisable, wherever possible, to obtain consent to perform hysterectomy should this become necessary. Again, pregnancy must be excluded.

Post-operative haematomata in the uterus are not uncommon and may give rise to ileus and, if infection occurs, the patient may have a very stormy course.

The usual post-operative stay is 7–10 days and the follow-up visit is six weeks after the operation.

Oophorectomy/ovarian cystectomy

A specimen of clotted blood should be sent for 'group and save serum'. If both ovaries are to be removed, it is usual to remove the uterus at the same time to prevent the possibility of uterine problems (particularly neoplasia) at a later date.

The usual post-operative stay is 4–10 days and the follow-up visit is six weeks after the operation; thereafter this depends on the indication for the operation and the histology.

Ventrosuspension

This is not very often performed these days, unless as part of another operation such as tubal surgery or myomectomy, and in certain cases of deep dyspareunia (see p. 41).

The usual post-operative stay is 3–7 days and the follow-up visit is usually 4–6 weeks after the operation.

Sterilisation

The husband's consent is usually required although the legal validity of this claim has yet to be tested in a court of law. The proposed technique needs to be explained clearly, reminding the patient that it is meant to be a definitive procedure and not a temporary alternative to contraception. It is essential to advise the patient that, whatever method used, there is a slight risk of failure. Pregnancy should again be excluded.

The usual post-operative stay depends on the technique employed but varies from one to seven days. The follow-up can be done by the G.P.

Hysterotomy

Two units of whole blood should be cross-matched and the Rhesus factor checked, as anti-D gammaglobulin may be required.

The usual post-operative stay is 5–10 days and the follow-up is usually six weeks after the operation. Ensure that the patient receives contraceptive advice and counsel her not to have another pregnancy for *at least* six months.

Laparoscopy

Cross-matching is not necessary. The usual post-operative stay varies from a day case to three days. The follow-up depends on the indication for the procedure and the findings.

Absolute contra-indications to laparoscopy are: severe cardiac disease, severe respiratory disease, and a history of generalised peritonitis and adhesions (especially if there are multiple abdominal scars). *Relative contra-indications* to laparoscopy are: obesity and a sub-umbilical laparotomy scar.

Vaginal Procedures

Dilatation and curettage (D & C)

You should check the patient's last menstrual period to ensure that, firstly, she is not pregnant, secondly, that it is the correct phase of the cycle if the investigation is for infertility, and thirdly, that she still has the symptoms for which the operation was advised — if there is a lengthy waiting list, a patient may have become menopausal or the original problem may have resolved.

The usual stay in hospital is rarely more than one day. The follow-up depends on the indications: the patient may need to be seen within two weeks for the histology results or in three months if the periods were irregular.

Evacuation of uterus

The Rhesus factor needs to be checked because anti-D gammaglobulin will be required if the patient is Rhesus negative. If the patient is pyrexial before operation, the procedure should be covered with antibiotics.

The usual stay in hospital is one day and follow-up can normally be done by the G.P. in six weeks. It may be necessary, in cases of recurrent miscarriage, to see the patient in the clinic in six weeks.

Termination of pregnancy

The Rhesus factor needs to be checked and blood sent for 'group and save serum'.

A very careful explanation of the type of therapeutic abortion (which is usually performed vaginally if less than 13 weeks gestation) should be given to the patient. The risks and dangers of abortion should have been explained to her by the gynaecologist who has agreed to, or recommended that, termination be performed. However, this should be checked before consent is obtained. It is important, in mid-trimester cases, to ensure that the patient is aware she may experience colicky abdominal pains similar to labour and that she will be conscious of the abortus at delivery. The possibility of further surgery, evacuation of the uterus, or rarely hysterotomy, must also be mentioned to the patient.

The duration of stay in hospital depends on the type of termination carried out, ranging from a day case in early vacuum aspirations to one week for hysterotomies.

Cone biopsy

A specimen of clotted blood should be sent for 'group and save serum'. The usual stay depends on the views of the surgeon and ranges from 2 to 14 days (in case there may be a secondary haemorrhage).

The follow-up visit to the out-patient clinic is two weeks later for results of the histology and thereafter depends on the histological findings.

Colporrhaphy and Manchester repair

A specimen of clotted blood should be sent for 'group and save serum'. The patient needs to be carefully watched for urinary retention if no catheter has been left in. If a pack is inserted, it is usually removed the day after operation.

The usual post-operative stay is 7–10 days and the follow-up visit is six weeks later.

Vaginal hysterectomy

The management is similar to that as for Manchester repair, but two units of whole blood should be cross-matched. Vault haematomata are a common complication of this surgery, so blood transfusion in the post-operative period may be necessary.

Post-operative Management

General points

It should be appreciated that there is a very wide variation in individual practice with regard to many aspects of post-operative management such as mobilisation, use of packs or drains, time of removal of drains, suture removal, duration of stay in hospital, and arrangements for follow-up. The above notes are meant as an approximate guide only and assume a fit patient without major post-operative complications. The ward Sister is the best person to ask about the management policies affecting patients on her ward. She can be your greatest ally and it should be remembered that she often knows more about the post-operative care of patients than the medical staff.

Finally, it should be remembered that, in addition to any specific complications related to the particular operation performed, the patient is still at risk of the several potential complications (e.g. chest infection or drug allergies) that may follow *any* operation and anaesthesia.

Recovery

Following any operation the patient will wish to know when she can: resume normal daily activities; resume intercourse, and return to work.

There is a very wide individual variation in patient's recovery from operation and therefore no hard-and-fast rules apply. The patient's G.P. is in the best position to give her guidance as he is likely to know her domestic circumstances better than the hospital doctors. However, in general terms, advice may be given to the patients as follows:

Minor procedures (e.g. laparoscopy, D & C, termination of pregnancy, cautery to cervix)

The patient should be recovered within a few days and back to normal in all respects in under a week; indeed many of these procedures are performed as day cases.

Intermediate procedures (e.g. sterilisation, cone biopsy, ventrosuspension)

The wounds will be healed within two weeks and the patient back to normal within four weeks. Many patients are fully recovered and able to return to full activity within two weeks.

Major procedures

Although the wounds will be healed within two weeks, the constitutional effects are much more marked. Despite feeling well, the patient tires easily and tends to overdo things initially. Whilst not encouraging a feeling of invalidism or wishing to recall the slow recuperation of yesteryear, it is usual for the patient to wait until after her six week follow-up clinic appointment before returning to full activity and work. There is no medical reason why a patient cannot return to work earlier but most welcome the opportunity of a rest. As regards resuming intercourse, most patients are afraid of 'damaging the operation' or anticipate that it will be painful. Such fears should be dispelled before they leave the ward. Once the wounds have healed, there is no reason why intercourse should not be gently resumed. Again most patient's prefer to wait for their postoperative check for confirmation that all is well. Patients are recommended not to resume driving a car until they are fully recovered from the immediate effects of surgery. This means that they are usually completely mobile and back to a normal, quiet, daily routine within four weeks of the operation.

Patients who have undergone radical and extensive operations will take longer to recover and their recovery is to a large extent governed by their attitudes, will-power, and the nature of the disorder for which the operation was performed.

Recovery is also often delayed in the elderly or those who suffer post-operative complications.

Out patient clinic

With the existing work load on the clinics, it is often necessary for the senior house officer to see follow-up patients and, although advice is readily available, it is useful to have some idea of which patients may be discharged from the clinic and which should be brought back. The recommendations listed below are guide lines for the beginner.

1. Patients who should *never* be discharged: those who have had treatment of a malignant disease, and those with a history of carcinoma in-situ.
2. Patients who *should* be brought back: those with abnormal cervical cytology, and those who are in a programme of investigations, e.g. amenorrhoea, infertility, urinary problems, or irregular menstruation.
3. Patients who *may* be discharged after confirming that the presenting symptoms have been treated satisfactorily; that the wound, if any, is soundly healed; that histology is satisfactory, *and* they have had *all* their queries answered and understand what has been done: those who have undergone abortion, sterilisation, hysterectomy for a benign lesion, ventrosuspension, colporrhaphies. Those who have successfully completed a programme of investigations and treatment, vaginal discharges and coil checks.

In many units patients who have undergone minor surgical procedures (such as sterilisation, evacuation of retained products, and polypectomy), are referred to their family practitioner for post-operative follow-up.

Index

A

abdominal operations
  hysterectomy 110
  hysterotomy 111
  laparoscopy 111–12
  myomectomy 110
  oophorectomy/ovarian
    cystectomy 110–11
  sterilisation 111
  ventrosuspension 111
abortion
  chromosomal factors 15
  definition 11
  examination 12
  habitual 14, 83
  history 11
  management 12–14
  maternal factors 14
  missed 13
  procedure 113–14
  symptoms and signs 6t
  therapeutic 113–14
  uterine factors 14–15
adenomyosis 22
alimentary symptoms 2
amenorrhoea
  bromocryptine 26–7
  examination 25–6
  follicle stimulating hormone
    (FSH) 26
  history 25
  hyperprolactinaemia 26–7
  hypothyroidism 26
  post-pill 28
  progesterone challenge 27, 28
anovulatory bleeding 78
antibiotics 87–8

anti-fungal agents
  clotrimazole 89
  miconazole 89–90
  nystatin 89
Asherman's syndrome 27

B

benign vulvitis 46
bimanual examination 3–4, 12, 26
  in abortion 12
  in amenorrhoea 26
bleeding
  dysfunctional 33–5, 77–8
  gynaecological
    emergencies 5–7
  see also menstruation, post
    menopausal bleeding
bromocryptine
  dosage 91
  indications 91
  in amenorrhoea 26–7
  side-effects 91

C

Candida albicans 45
  see also Monilia
carcinoma
  cervical 55, 57, 59
  endometrial 31, 82
  ovarian 22, 23
  vulval 45–6, 47
cervical cytology, abnormal
  histology 58

cervical cytology (*continued*)
  intra-epithelial neoplasia *see* Cervical Intra-epithelial Neoplasia(CIN)
  smears 57–8
  terminology 55, 56t, 57
cervical excitation 6t, 7, 17–8
Cervical Intra-epithelial Neoplasia(CIN)
  management 59
  terminology 55, 56t, 57
cervical smears
  abnormal 55, 57–8
  procedure 53
chemical spermicides 99
cholelithiasis 105
cholecystitis 105
chromosomal factors in abortion 15
climacteric
  hormone replacement therapy 84–5
  symptoms 84
clomiphene
  dosage 92–3
  indications 92–3
  in male subfertility 68
coil 99–100
colporrhaphy 114
colposcopy 57–8
condom 98
cone biopsy 58, 114
congestive dysmenorrhoea 37–8
contraception
  chemical spermicides 99
  condom 98
  intra-uterine devices 99–100
  occlusive caps 99
  rhythm method 97–8
  withdrawal methods 98
  see also oral contraceptives
curettage
  diagnostic 29
  and dilatation *see* dilatation and curettage
cystic hyperplasia 30, 34
cytology
  genital tract 53–4
  see also cervical cytology

D

deep dyspareunia 41–2
detrusor instability 72
dilatation and curettage (D&C) 113
dysfunctional bleeding
  examination 33
  history 33
  hormone therapy 77–8
  management 33–4
dysmenorrhoea
  congestive 37–8
  endometriosis 38, 39
  examination 37
  history 37
  hormone therapy 78–9
  and pelvic infection 38
  spasmodic 37–8
dyspareunia
  deep 41–2
  history 41
  superficial 41
dysplasia 55, 56t

E

ectopic pregnancy
  diagnosis 5, 7
  symptoms and signs 6t
emergencies
  rectal examination 7
  surgical conditions 5
  symptoms and signs 6t
  tubal pregnancy 5
  vaginal examination 7
endocervical smear 53
endometrial smear 53
endometriosis
  and dysmenorrhoea 38, 39
  hormone therapy 79
  internal 22
epimenorrhagia 77
epimenorrhoea 77
erosion 51, 52
examination 3–4

F

female genital tract,
  cytology 53–4
  see also smears
fertility drugs
  bromocryptine 91
  clomiphene 92–3
  gonadotrophins 93
  tamoxifen 93
fibroids 22
follicle stimulating hormone (FSH)
  and amenorrhoea 26
  as fertility drug 93
  in male subfertility 66

G

generalised pruritus 43, 45
genital tract cytology 53–4
gonadotrophins
  as fertility drugs 93
  see also follicle stimulating
    hormone, luteinising hormone
gynaecological examination 3–4

H

habitual abortion 14, 83
heavy menstruation
  examination 33
  history 33
  management 33–4, 77–8
history-taking
  menstrual 1–2
  obstetric 2
hormone preparations
  danazol 80–1
  dydrogesterone 80
  norethisterone 80
hormone replacement
  therapy 84–5
hormone therapy
  dysfunctional bleeding 33–4,
    77–8
  dysmenorrhoea 78–9
  endometrial carcinoma 82
  endometriosis 79
  premenstrual syndrome 79
  subfertility 67–8
  see also climacteric symptoms
human menopausal
  gonadotrophin 93
hyperplasia
  adenomatous 30, 34
  cystic 30, 34
hyperprolactinaemia
  and amenorrhoea 26–7
  bromocriptine therapy 91
  in male subfertility 66
hypertension, and oral
  contraceptives 103, 105
hypothyroidism, and
  amenorrhoea 26
hysterectomy
  dysfunctional bleeding 34
  procedure 110
  vaginal 114
hysterotomy 111

I

incontinence see urinary
  incontinence
internal endometriosis 22
intra-uterine devices 99–100
irregular menstruation
  examination 33
  history 33
  management 33–4

L

Lactobacillus acidophilus 51
laparoscopy
  contraindications 112
  in dysmenorrhoea 37
  in pelvic pain 18
  procedure 111–12
lateral wall vaginal smear 53–4
luteinising hormone (LH)
  as fertility drug 93
  in amenorrhoea 26
  in endometriosis 79
  in male subfertility 66

localised pruritus 45–6
low back pain 19

M

malignant curettings 31
Manchester repair 114
maternal factors, in abortion 14
menopause, hormone replacement therapy 84–5
menstrual history 1–2
menstruation
   see irregular menstruation, heavy menstruation
miscarriage 11
missed abortion 11, 13
Monilia 50, 51, 57, 89
myomectomy 110

N

neoplasia see carcinoma

O

obstetric history 2
occlusive caps 99
oestrogen–progesterone contraceptives
   contraindications 101–3
   effects on bleeding 104
   side-effects 103–4
   surgery and 104–5
oestrogens
   for climacteric symptoms 84–5
   for dysfunctional bleeding 33–4, 77–8
oophorectomy 110–11
operations
   practical aspects 109
   see also abdominal operations, vaginal operations
oral contraceptives 101–7
   drug interactions 104t
   failure 105
   monitoring of patients 105
   see also oestrogen–progesterone contraceptives
   progestogen-only preparations 106
   side-effects
      cholecystitis and cholelithiasis 105
      hypertension 106
      stroke 105
      thrombo-embolism 106
ovarian accidents 6t
ovarian cystectomy 110–11
ovarian masses 22–3
ovular bleeding 77–8
ovulation, and subfertility 62
oxytocics 94–5

P

Paget's disease 46
pain 5–7, 17, 18
   abdomino-pelvic 5–7
   shoulder tip 17, 18
   see also low back pain, pelvic pain
pelvic examination 3–4
pelvic infection
   dysmenorrhoea and 38
   symptoms and signs 6t
pelvic masses
   examination 21
   history 21
   ovarian 22–3
   tubo-ovarian 23
   uterine 22
pelvic pain
   examination 17–8
   history 17
   management 18
   syndrome 18
post-coital test 62
post menopausal bleeding (PMB)
   examination 29
   history 29
   management 29–31
post-operative management
   general points 115
   out patient clinic 117
   recovery 115–17

Index

pregnancy
  termination of 113–14
  see also tubal pregnancy
premenstrual syndrome 79
progesterone challenge 27–8
progestogen-only
    contraceptives 106
progestogens
  in dysfunctional
    bleeding 33–4, 78
  in endometrial carcinoma 82
  in habitual abortion 83
prolactin
  in amenorrhoea 26
  in subfertility 63
prostaglandins 95
pruritus vulvae 43–7
  generalised 43–4
  localised 45–6
Pseudomonas pyocyanea 87
psychological factors
  in dyspareunia 41
  in pelvic pain 18
  in subfertility 63

R

rectal examination 4, 7
Rhesus factor, in abortion 12
rhythm method 97–8

S

safe period 97–8
salpingitis 18
Schiller's test 57–8
semen
  analysis 61–2
  characteristics 65–6
shoulder tip pain 17, 18
smears
  endocervical 53
  endometrial 53
  lateral wall vaginal 53
  vaginal 53–4
  see also cervical smears
spasmodic dysmenorrhoea
  management 38
  occurrence 37

spermicides 99
sterilisation 111
stress incontinence
  symptoms 69–70
  treatment 73–4
  urodynamic studies 72
stroke, and oral
    contraceptives 105
subfertility
  female 61–3
    examination 61
    history 61
    ovulation 62
    post coital test 62
    prolactin levels 63
    semen analysis 61–2
    tubal patency 62
  male 65–8
    examination 65
    history 65
    hormone assays 66
    investigations 65–7
    testicular biopsy 67
    therapy 67–8
superficial dyspareunia 41
surgery *see* operations

T

testicular biopsy 67
therapeutic abortion 113–14
thrombo-embolism, and oral
    contraceptives 101, 105
thyroid function test
  in amenorrhoea 26
  in subfertility 63
Trichomonas vaginalis
  abnormal cervical cytology
    and 57
  in vaginal discharge 45, 49, 50
  treatment 50, 88, 89
true incontinence 69
tubal patency 62
tubal pregnancy
  diagnosis 5, 7
  signs and symptoms 6t
tubo-ovarian masses 23

U

urge incontinence 70
urinary incontinence
  management 72–4
  neurological examination 71
  pelvic examination 71
  true 69
  urge 70
  see also stress incontinence
urodynamic studies 72
uterine mass 22
uterine muscle stimulants
  ergometrine 94
  oxytocin 94
  prostaglandins 95
uterus
  and abortion 14–15
  enlarged 33
  evacuation of 113
  retroverted 42

V

vaginal bleeding *see* bleeding
vaginal discharge
  examination 50
  history 49
  in pruritus vulvae 43, 45
  management 50–1
vaginal operations
  colporrhaphy and Manchester repair 114
  cone biopsy 114
  dilatation and curettage 113
  evacuation of the uterus 113
  termination of pregnancy 113–14
  vaginal hysterectomy 114
vaginal swabs 50
vaginismus 41
ventrosuspension 111
vulva 3, 45–6
  dystrophic changes 45–6
  visible changes 45
  see also pruritus vulvae
vulvectomy 46, 47

W

withdrawal methods 98